Sex, Frankly

Sex, Frankly
What Couples, Singles, Teens, and Parents Want To Know

Marshall L. Shearer, MD
Marguerite R. Shearer, MD

Edited by Stephen Geez

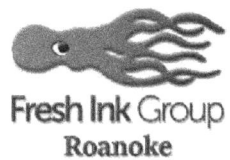

Fresh Ink Group
Roanoke

Sex, Frankly
What Teens, Singles, Couples, And Parents Want To Know

Copyright © 1972, 2012, 2016
Marshall L. Shearer, MD
Marguerite R. Shearer, MD
Editor: Stephen Geez

Fresh Ink Group
An Imprint of:
The Fresh Ink Group, LLC
PO Box 525
Roanoke, TX 76262
Email: info@FreshInkGroup.com
www.FreshInkGroup.com

Edition 1.0   2012
Edition 1.1   2016

Book design by Ann E. Stewart
Cover design by Stephen Geez
Cover layout by Janet Shelby

Except as permitted under the U.S. Copyright Act of 1976, no part of this publication may be reproduced, distributed, or transmitted in any form or by any means, or stored in a database or retrieval system, without prior written permission of the publisher.

Cataloging-in-Publication Recommendations: Sex (Non-Fiction);
Sex Education (Non-Fiction); Relationships (Non-Fiction);
Sex Therapy (Non-Fiction); Pregnancy (Non-Fiction); Contraception (Non-Fiction);
Health (Non-Fiction); STDs (Non-Fiction); Marriage (Non-Fiction);
Childhood Development (Non-Fiction)

Library of Congress Control Number: 2011937932

ISBN: 978-1-936442-09-6

*Dedicated to the principle
that a morality based on fear or ignorance
is no morality at all*

Table of Contents

1. Introduction 1

2. **What People Call Love** 3
   Negative Attention 3
   Positive Attention 3
   Opportunity To Give 4
   Altruism 4
   Acceptance 5
   Admiration 5
   Respect 6
   "Understand Me" and "Believe in Me" 6
   Our Definition of Love 7
   Love Versus Infatuation 7
   Object of Dating 7

3. **Sexual Intercourse: Arousal to Afterglow** 9
   Arousal Differences 9
   Erogenous Body Zones 10
   Petting Techniques 11
   The Effects of Arousal 11
   Oral Sex 12
   The Thrusting Motion 12
   The Orgasm 12
   The Afterglow 13
   Insertion of the Penis 14
   Duration of Intercourse 14
   After Intercourse 15
   Semen in the Vagina 15

4. **Positions for Sexual Intercourse** 17
   Natural Position 17
   Most Common Position 17
   Rear-Entry Position 18
   Astride Position 18
   Side Position 18
   The Best Position? 19
   Position and Pregnancy 19

5. First Intercourse 21
Virginity and the Hymen 21
Discomfort During First Intercourse 21
The Position 22
Nudity 23

6. Sex Before Long-term Commitment 25
Setting for Premarital Intercourse 25
Reasons for Pre-relationship Intercourse 26
Curiosity 26
Peer Pressure 27
Inability to Set Limits 27
Proof of Sexual Adequacy 28
To Hold On to the Man 29
Expression of Anger 30
Just Pleasure 31
To Give Unselfishly of Self 32
Carried Away by Emotions 33
Expression of Intimacy 33
Expression of Love 34
Effects on Married Life 34
Effects on Love 36
To Make Love Complete 37
Marriage 37
Partner's History 38
Considerations Prior to Premarital Intercourse 38
"Backing Up" 39
Self-control 40

7. Ambivalence and the Sex Act 43
Frigidity 43
Frigid or Clumsy 43
Lack of Sex Instruction 44
Sex Without Orgasm 45
Love Without Sex 47
Penis Size and Frigidity 49
Physical Incompatibility of Genitalia 49
Communication and Relationship 50
Importance of Anger 51
Premature Ejaculation 51
Delayed Ejaculation 52
Impotence 52

8. Incompatibility: Physical and Psychological 55
Size of the Vagina 55
Size of the Penis 55
Psychological Incompatibility 56

9. Intimacy Without Intercourse 59
Growth of a Relationship 59
Transcultural Misunderstanding 59
Sexual Reputations 60
Turning On 61
Setting Limits 62
Petting Without Intercourse 62
Orgasm Without Intercourse 63

10. Masturbation 65
Physical Effects of Masturbation 65
Thoughts While Masturbating 65
Guilt 66
Female Masturbation 67
Nocturnal Emission 68

11. Feeling, Thinking, and Doing 69
Sexual Feelings Only 70
Prostitute-relationship 70
The Other Extreme 71
Rapists 71
Nymphomaniacs 71
Perversions 72
Homosexuality 73
Oral-genital Contact 76

12. Menstruation 79
The Menstrual Cycle 79
Arousal at the Time of Ovulation 79
Premenstrual Tension 80
Intercourse During Menstruation 81
Onset of Menstruation 81

13. Contraception 83
A Basis for Comparison 83
The Douche 83
The Rhythm Method 83

    Basal Temperature 84
    Coitus Interruptus 85
    The Diaphragm 85
    Intravaginal Preparations 86
    The Condom 86
    Combo 87
    The Intrauterine Contraceptive Device 87
    The Pill 88
    The "Morning-after Pill" 90
    The Sterilization Operation 91
    A Summary of Contraception 92

14. Pregnancy and Alternatives to Parenthood 95
    Signs of Pregnancy 95
    Seeing the Doctor 95
    Options with Pregnancy 96
    Adoption 96
    Keeping the Baby 97
    Placement of the Baby 97

15. Abortion 99
    Abortion 99
    Reasons for an Abortion 100
    Illegal Abortion 100
    Psychological Effects of Illegal Abortion 101
    The Abortion Debate 102
    Role of Religion in Society 102
    Rights of Society 103
    Rights of the Fetus 105
    Rights of Women 108
    Laws to Enforce Morals 109

16. Sexually Transmitted Disease 111
    Sexually Transmitted Disease 111
    Syphilis 112
    Gonorrhea 113
    Chlamydia 113
    HIV/AIDS 113
    HPV/Genital Warts 114
    Herpes 114
    Crabs and Scabies 114
    Avoiding STDs 115

17. Marriage 117
Premarital Exam 117
Douching 117
Honeymoon Cystitis 117
Rules and Regulations of Marriage 118
Frequency of Intercourse in Marriage 119
Sexual Compatibility 120
"Cooling" with Time 121
Extramarital Affairs 122
Intercourse and Pregnancy 123
Effects of Aging in Men 123
Erectile Dysfunction 124
Testicle Exam 125
Effects of Aging in Women 126
Breast Exam 127

18. Parenting and Child Sexual Development 129
Early Childhood 129
Age Two to Six 130
Concepts of Death 134
Sexual Feelings 134
Masturbation 135
Sexual Roles 136
Sexual Curiosity 139
Age Eight to Ten 139
Interest in Sexual Materials 140
Menstrual Education 141
Nocturnal Emissions 142
Normal Homosexual Attachments 144
Homosexual Activity 144
Conditions For Homosexuality 145
Seductive Behavior with a Child 145
Influences 147

19. About the Authors: 149

Introduction

For two years the Shearers accepted invitations to talk about sex with groups of 100-200 housing-unit residents on the campus of the University of Michigan. Later the university administration began sponsoring the wildly popular discussions, and the groups swelled to as many as 2,000 each. Participants were free to submit anonymous questions in advance, plus ask anything they wanted in person, no topic too risqué, all subjects allowed. Material from those presentations first appeared in the Shearers' book *Rapping About Sex...* way back in 1972.

Since then, the Shearers have worked with thousands of patients—she in family medicine, he in psychiatry and couples therapy, together at the Masters and Johnson Institute—and educated millions through their books and syndicated "Sex Help" column appearing for 23 years in major newspapers. Throughout it all they noticed something very poignant: Even as medicine and technology advance, the essence of people's questions remains the same.

Sex, Frankly builds on those original meetings, then expands the discussion to include everyone from curious teens to loving parents raising healthy, happy children. What *has* changed is popular media. Subjects once avoided or handled discreetly are now "in your face," but any glut of information brings misinformation, assumptions and myths, expectations and disappointments.

Sex, Frankly cuts through it all with the simple, unvarnished truth. It deals with real questions from real people living in the real world. It's everyone's private conversation with the experts. Any time is a good time to learn, and this book is the best place to start because, frankly, it's all about sex.

Chapter 1
What People Call Love

PEG: Many who are engaging in sexual intercourse consider themselves in love. The question then becomes, What is their definition of love? One's concept of love is individually determined. It is essentially the best (the most psychologically satisfying) interpersonal relationship one has ever experienced.

Negative Attention

Some people will settle simply for negative attention as love. If nobody paid sufficient attention to them when they were young, they often learn to settle for any kind of attention, including negative attention or even abusive attention. Emotional neglect can occur in every socio-economic class. Some parents cannot give; they have never been given to and do not know how. Others do not give for egocentric, selfish reasons. Still other parents place a higher value on some other endeavors. They are not aware of the price they and their children pay for a barren, emotional climate. Children from these families will usually settle for any kind of attention, even negative attention, especially if the most meaningful attention they got from their parents had been negative attention; that is, they could always get their parents' attention by "being bad" and seldom by "being good." It might well be better to be abused than to be ignored.

Positive Attention

There are those who settle for positive attention: occasional contact, casual outings, social networking. "No one ever paid that much attention to me before; it's wonderful." Maybe it is inexperienced love, but maybe it is escape from loneliness and the most anybody would do.

Opportunity To Give

MARSHALL: There are others who will call the opportunity to give, love. They operate on a "use me" basis: "I have never been considered worth enough to have anything to give to anybody else. No one has said you have something to give; you can make a contribution. No one has ever asked of me."

Altruism

These kids are from good, middle-class, materialistic homes where they have all the conveniences. They have never been made responsible for any part of it. Any job is easier to do yourself than letting a child do it initially, but never asking something of a child may create a serious inferiority complex in him or her. In these families, the child's job has been to go to school, do the best he can (for his own sake), and perhaps clean his room. High-school and college age tend to be the most idealistic of any ages in life. It is natural to want to give. It is laudable to want to be unselfish. For many of these adolescents and young adults, especially for young ladies, the first time they are really asked to give is to give happiness by giving of their body. They may well call this being in love. But, if the relationship does not grow, what they are settling for is reciprocated gratitude in place of love. In the extreme this reaches the proportions of the "kept lover," man or woman, who is supported financially and sexually.

Of course, the need to give and be altruistic can be exploited by either party, and in either direction. One twist is a man outside of the mainstream challenging a woman to prove she is not biased by having intercourse with him. A surprising number of women accept this challenge and have intercourse for no other reason.

Exploitation in the other direction generates feelings of superiority. It is not limited just to sex. It can occur on more sophisticated levels, with domination being love given, and gratitude and dependency being love returned. It may be exploitation by the male as well as the female. For example, "Let me teach you something, you poor ignorant you." It can also occur on a more global level: "Let me introduce you to the finer things in life (fine arts), you poor peasant you." (This is the basis for some marriages between people of an entirely different social class.) Or, "Let me marry you and support you financially through school, you pauper you." Eventually they break up, and she wonders why. Maybe he needed a chance to give a little, too, and she still needs to play mama. She might call him "ungrateful," as though if he continued to be grateful and dependent it would still be "love."

<u>Acceptance</u>

This next concept of love is "accept me." "Accept me for the person I am. Don't hassle me. Take me or leave me." You can imagine their family backgrounds. Nothing is ever wholly right. Make four *A's* and one *B* and all you hear about is that *B*. To really feel you measure up to someone else's expectations, to be accepted as you are, without being asked to change this or that about yourself, can be pretty great—and may be confused with love.

<u>Admiration</u>

PEG: Others will settle for admiration and call this love. Their backgrounds are pretty similar in many ways to those who settle for acceptance. They have never been in the limelight, never had much prestige, never made any team, let alone been popular. If you have never been looked up to, you are likely to call it love the first time it happens. Gifts, favors, and attention can go awfully far along this line. Ever been on a pedestal before, even a little one? Ever been center stage, just for being you?

MARSHALL: Pretended admiration is one way young men may consciously deceive young ladies, and occasionally vice versa.

Respect

Before we give our definition of love, there is another dimension to consider: *respect.* You need to be able to respect the other person, respect his or her opinions, values, and feelings, and respect him or her as an individual. You should be able to respect the other person's feelings about sexual activity just as you would respect his or her feelings about smoking or drinking. Whether you are male or female, you should expect to receive respect for your feelings and your values. This does not mean they should not be discussed; they should, and each of you will need to convey the depth of your feelings and convictions. You will want to reconsider at your own leisure those values which are questioned by the person you love, but remember in love your feelings and values are not something that have to be analyzed away, or things that have to be justified. They are part of you. You are what you feel, what you believe in. Love presumes acceptance and respect of you and what you believe.

"Understand Me" and "Believe in Me"

The two other steps in this dimension, "understand me" and "believe in me," are not prerequisites for love. They grow as the love grows. To what extent are you going to believe in your partner if, for example, he or she quits a good job on principle? You probably can accept and respect the decision, and that is enough for love, but will you, can you, understand why your partner considered it so important? Furthermore, will you continue to believe in the one you love?

Our Definition of Love

Love is caring equally as much about the other person's happiness as you care about your own. In some moments, love should be caring more about the other person's happiness than your own. That is fine and good; soldiers earn medals in combat for that, which is fine, but that is easy compared to really caring about the little things, the things of every day, day-in, day-out, week after week, year after year.

Love Versus Infatuation

Is there any way you can differentiate feelings of love from sexual attraction?

MARSHALL: I cannot give you any short or quick answer. I think that time would prove which it is. I think that a sharing of hopes and fears and sadnesses and happinesses would be part of it. Really, you commit to someone with whom you can relate on many levels, someone you can trust and trust to love you. This is one of the advantages of dating, pre-marital engagement periods, or cohabiting.

PEG: Use your head and think about your potential partner. What attracts you? Thought is a substitute for trial action. This, of course, does not mean that you go around over-analyzing all your relationships. Lead with your heart, not your head; but at some point in a relationship, whether it is marriage or premarital intercourse, stop and use your head to decide if you should give your heart full play.

Object of Dating

This does not mean that every time you go out with somebody of the opposite sex you should do so with the idea of potential sex or marriage. If that is the only reason you date, you are going to have a lot of disappointments. Go out just for fun, for a change of scenery. Have fun together and let your heart, your hearts, take the lead and set the pace. Then use your head to set the direction and distance you want to go together.

Chapter 2
Sexual Intercourse: Arousal to Afterglow

Arousal Differences

MARSHALL: We get a lot of questions about intercourse, including the basic: How do you go about it? So let us start with *arousal*. Women and men are different psychologically, as well as anatomically, in what arouses them. If you look at content targeted for males, you will see that many of the pictures focus on the woman's body and suggestive poses. This kind of thing can be quite exciting to a man. A man can get excited just by thinking about it. Whereas, if you look at women's content where a picture is supposed to have sexual connotations, you will see smartly dressed people, well-decorated rooms; there is an atmosphere, a mood. This example typifies the major difference between what psychologically stimulates men and what psychologically stimulates women.

Somehow it always comes as a shock to young adolescent boys to find out that girls are not aroused simply by the sight of male bodies. Now, this aspect of what arouses women has some implications for the development of the race; namely, this feeling of being cared for, this atmosphere, is a guarantee, a biological guarantee, that the man with whom she has intercourse will care about her, will help take care of her and the child when it is born. Of course, the very fact that the man can watch a pretty lady at a distance and get stimulated by looking may have something to say for the survival of the race, too. A man may also be attracted at a distance by the sight of suggestive clothing, the sound of a feminine voice, or by the aroma of perfume. Of course sight, sound, and smell are also important to the woman, but chiefly as they contribute to the mood and atmosphere.

So there are sexual differences in which mode of sexual attraction predominates in the very early stage. This difference persists to a lesser degree throughout the act of intercourse. It accounts for the fact that generally men prefer to have intercourse in a well-lighted area, increasing their sexual stimulation by looking, while the woman often prefers a quasi-dark room with its atmosphere. It accounts for the fact that a man can have intercourse most anywhere, while many women cannot become aroused unless the place and atmosphere are "right." It further contributes to the difference in distractibility during intercourse. The attraction stage is followed by sexual arousal through physical contact such as cuddling, hugging, and kissing (touch and taste, if you will).

Erogenous Body Zones

An erogenous zone is an area of the body that when stimulated increases sexual excitement. These include the genitals themselves: in the man, the penis; and in the woman, the vagina, the external genitalia, and particularly the organ called the clitoris, which is just forward of the outlet of the bladder. At least in our society, the mouth's lips and tongue are erogenous zones in both sexes, and the usual stimulation is kissing. In women, the breasts are an erogenous zone, also; however, there are some women who are "turned off" by breast stimulation. The lobe of the ear, the area of the buttocks, and the anus itself are erogenous in some individuals, both men and women. Petting involves stimulation in any of the erogenous areas. Actually, any area of the body may be stimulating when caressed.

For the best arousal in lovemaking, there must be free communication between the couple regarding which zone they might get the greatest excitement from at that moment, and whether the stimulation is too hard, too light, too fast, or too slow, etc. Nonverbal communication is usually preferable, as it can be more spontaneous and less distracting.

Petting Techniques

What is fingering?

Fingering, fondling, "hand job," and many slang terms refer to the man using his hands to stimulate and caress the woman's external genitalia, or perhaps placing a finger in the vagina; and the woman caressing the man's penis with her hands. Again, stimulation can be too hard or too light for a given individual, so this information should be freely communicated. In general, moist friction is stimulating while dry friction is irritating, especially to women.

The Effects of Arousal

In the male, sexual excitement produces an erect penis. The penis becomes erect ("stands up") and becomes hard because the veins that drain the blood away from the penis clamp down. The arteries or the vessels that bring blood into the penis open up, and the penis enlarges and becomes stiff, just as a garden hose will straighten out if the nozzle is closed and the faucet is fully opened.

In the female, the corresponding process of sexual arousal is a secretion from the walls of the vagina which acts as a lubricant during intercourse. The female usually lubricates with physical contact, but just as the male may have an erection without petting, the female may become sexually aroused and lubricate without petting. If the proceedings do not go on to intercourse, the woman may notice some discharge from the vagina, and the man may notice a drop or two of lubricating secretion from the penis. Women who are not adequately aroused prior to the insertion of the penis and do not have adequate lubrication usually need more time and stimulation, and they should say so.

Oral Sex

Oral sex involves using the mouth to stimulate a sex partner's genitals. Stimulating a penis is called *fellatio*, a "blow job," and many other slang terms. Stimulating a woman's genitals, usually emphasizing the clitoris, is called *cunnilingus* and many slang terms. Some people are turned off by the very idea. Some use it as the complete sex act to achieve orgasm, perhaps because circumstances make it easier, to avoid risk of pregnancy, to preserve "virginity," or to save intercourse for a time of greater commitment. Some use oral-genital contact as part of the pre-orgasmic arousal phase, or "foreplay."

The Thrusting Motion

After the arousal phase, the man inserts his penis into the vagina, partially withdrawing and reinserting it in an alternating, quasi-rhythmic motion. The woman may also thrust with her hips, and may even take the lead. Sexual excitement during the act of intercourse advances in plateaus, building up in a kind of steplike fashion, preferably in a mutually satisfying rhythm, to greater and greater intensities, greater and greater tension, to the point of orgasm.

The Orgasm

Orgasm in the male, physiologically speaking, is the release of fluid called semen from the penis, about 3 to 5 cubic centimeters or a teaspoonful. This fluid contains sperm, which in most men is capable of fertilizing an egg. The semen is propelled from the penis by rhythmic contractions of several muscles. In the female there is nothing physiologically comparable to the release of semen or fluid from the man's penis; however, the woman does have similar muscle contractions in the outer third of the vagina, and she may experience a rapid increase in lubrication. In both the man and the woman there is a psychological orgasm which is very similar, if not identical. Orgasm is one more heightening of sexual excitement or tension, one more step which is held only momentarily, a few seconds (slightly longer in women than men), and then this peak of sexual tension falls off. A woman may be multi-orgasmic; that is, she may have several orgasms, maintaining a high level of sexual excitement during the interval. A man may experience several orgasms in a day, but his body requires an interval between them of at least fifteen minutes and up to several hours.

The Afterglow

After the orgasm, there is complete relaxation, complete release from tension, complete relaxation of muscle tone. Often there is a feeling of oneness: a feeling of loss of identity as you become fused with your sex partner; a floating feeling; a complete feeling of contentment and fulfillment. This feeling trails off, dims out like a glowing coal dies out. This phase is called the afterglow. Some people do not value this phase of intercourse very much, but others regard it as the most valuable. Buddhism and Hinduism value the state of sexual afterglow. Particularly with people who are experiencing their first intercourse or engaging in acts beyond their comfort zones, there may be a period of depression shortly after the orgasm, say thirty seconds afterwards, due perhaps to guilt or unconscious doubts: "Have I been had?" "Was my body just used to masturbate with?" "Does he (or she) really care about me as a person?" "I thought that would be fun, but now I feel dirty." Such depression may occur after marriage as well as before. At times, this feeling may linger if not dealt with. A kiss might help dispel it. One partner "rolling over and going to sleep" while ignoring the other's feelings can make it worse.

Insertion of the Penis

How does a woman know when she is ready to receive the erect penis? On an average, how long does intercourse take?

PEG: The signs of being sufficiently aroused for insertion of the penis would be adequate vaginal lubrication and some different sensation in the pelvis, a sort of "pelvic awareness." Pelvic throbbing indicates greater arousal. After some experience in a trusting relationship, you will be able to judge from your psychic state; you will just know. This points up the importance of the relationship in the first experiences with intercourse.

Duration of Intercourse

MARSHALL: Although it varies widely from person to person and even occasion to occasion, on the average the thrusting phase lasts two to three minutes, and its duration is determined by several factors. The male's orgasm with his usual subsequent loss of erection determines the duration of intercourse. A woman may have several orgasms during a single episode of intercourse without her level of sexual excitement dropping very far. After an orgasm, a man can have a second erection within several minutes. The second intercourse, whether minutes, hours, or a day later, will usually last longer. Here the sexual response is following a standard biological law: the absolute and relative refractory periods. After an organ has responded, there is a period of time when it cannot make the response again. This is followed by another period of time during which it can only make the response with a greater than usual stimulus.

How soon a man will ejaculate is in turn dependent upon several factors. Generally speaking, the more recently the man has ejaculated, up to about three days, the longer intercourse will last. The higher the plateau of arousal on insertion into the vagina, the shorter the thrusting phase. Within some limits, the faster the rate of thrusting stimulation, the sooner orgasm will occur.

Psychological factors are equally or perhaps more important. If a man is goal-oriented—that is, driving for orgasm—he may not last as long as if he were savoring every moment. Also, his perception of his partner's involvement often is a major factor. He will have an orgasm more rapidly if he perceives she "is just doing it for him," or if he perceives she is in a hurry from fear of discovery or is thinking of her next customer if she is a prostitute. Some men develop premature ejaculation habits under such circumstances.

All this considered, the first intercourse is probably not going to last very long, perhaps only a few seconds. The woman will probably feel unfulfilled at this point. Hopefully, both will feel secure and free enough to continue some form of love play until she is satisfied.

After Intercourse

Is a man sterile right after intercourse?

PEG: No. He may not be able to have an erection for several minutes, but that is not sterility. His next ejaculation will contain sperm capable of causing pregnancy.

Semen in the Vagina

What happens to the liquid ejected by the man? Is it absorbed by the woman's body, gotten rid of through the vaginal opening, or what?

PEG: A portion of semen is absorbed through the vaginal lining, but the majority is probably just expelled through the vaginal opening.

Chapter 3
Positions for Sexual Intercourse

Natural Position

What are the positions for intercourse, and what is the most natural position according to anatomy?

MARSHALL: A natural position for sexual intercourse is one which is mutually acceptable, stimulating, and comfortable. The important factors of positions are: Where is the weight? Which body parts are free? Which partner is free to thrust? What kind and how much intimacy is desire? Are the partners seeking variety or acting out a fantasy?

Most Common Position

The most common position in our society is the woman on her back with the man between her legs facing her. This position has the advantage of face-to-face intimacy where two people can look each other in the eye and easily kiss. The disadvantages are that the woman must remain relatively inactive, is somewhat pinned, and bears more of the man's weight than in any other position. The psychological aspect of these disadvantages are often the critical factor. For a woman to relax and be spontaneous in this position requires a high degree of trust in her partner.

A variation of this position is with the woman remaining in the same position with the man's upper body being perpendicular to the bed. For example, the woman could lie on her back on the bed with the man standing on the floor between her legs. Since there is no weight on the abdomen, this position is used particularly during pregnancy.

Rear-Entry Position

With the rear-entry position, the woman bends at the hips and the man enters from behind. The couple may be standing, on their knees, lying on their sides, or with him sitting and her on his lap. This position allows less intimacy.

Astride Position

In another position the woman may be astride the man with him either sitting up or on his back. The woman is completely free of all the psychological accompaniments of having the male above her. She is in the best position to insert the penis (moving back onto it, not straight down on it). Often this degree of control of proceedings allays a great deal of fear in the relatively inexperienced woman. The woman also provides most or all of the motion. For variety, this position can be quite enjoyable for both male and female. It is especially advantageous when the man is physically tired, injured, handicapped, or has reason not to exert himself too much, such as after a heart attack.

Side Position

Masters and Johnson described a position in which either partner may set a thrusting pattern or both may thrust simultaneously. Neither partner is pinned down, each has one arm free, and there is minimal weight supported by the other. Unfortunately, the position is somewhat difficult to learn. The man can be on his back or any degree to his side with one hip and knee bent at a 90° angle and flat on the bed. The woman is astride his other leg with her side on a pillow on the bed above the man's bent thigh and against his body. Obviously the position will require some experimentation.

The Best Position?

Whatever position feels right and is most stimulating at the time is the best position. Be willing to explore and experiment. Different positions can add variety and zest to sexual intercourse.

Position and Pregnancy

As far as the position in which a woman is most likely to become pregnant, many authorities recommend that she lie on her back with her hips raised. The position in which a woman is least likely to become pregnant would be manual or oral-genital gratification without intercourse.

If a woman lies prostrate, is she more likely to get pregnant? Is it better for her to walk around if she is worried about getting pregnant?

PEG: Do not bank on it. It may be therapeutic for a woman who has difficulty getting pregnant to stay in bed and put a pillow under her hips, but to do the opposite as a method of contraception is wholly inadequate.

MARSHALL: Carry a condom and spermicide. They are not that expensive. And if you do not happen to have one, what is the big hurry that the two of you cannot postpone intercourse for as much as half an hour to get adequate protection? Condoms improvised out of bread wrappers or sandwich wrappers are not safe. Consider the risk. Consider the alternatives to pregnancy out of wedlock.

Chapter 4
First Intercourse

What about first intercourse? How should you do it?

Virginity and the Hymen

PEG: I think these questions on initial experiences with intercourse for the woman are primarily related to concerns about virginity and the hymen. The hymen is a membrane that covers the opening of the vagina. The hymen itself has a small opening in it, through which menstruation occurs. It can vary considerably in thickness from person to person, from tissue-paper thinness to the thickness of skin. By the same token, the opening in the membrane can vary a great deal. Some women have a very small opening while others have so large an opening that the hymen does not seem to exist.

If you are examined by a physician before intercourse (e.g., a premarital examination), the physician can give you some idea of the relative thickness of your hymen and the size of the opening, and can suggest how to reduce any difficulty he or she thinks you might have with initial intercourse. Occasionally, and this is not common, a woman will have a very thick hymen with a very small opening which would preclude sexual intercourse. This condition can be taken care of in a doctor's office with the very minor operative procedure of just making the opening larger so that intercourse would be feasible.

Discomfort During First Intercourse

The amount of bleeding that occurs at the first intercourse is related to the thickness of the hymen, the size of the opening, and whether blood vessels are torn during the dilatation of the opening. A thick hymen will have fair-sized blood vessels which, when torn, will bleed more than smaller blood vessels. So the amount of bleeding varies. Usually it is not a problem, and one should not be alarmed by a small amount of bleeding. There may be a single sharp pain when the hymen tears. It is usually not a severe pain and does not linger or recur.

The Position

What is the best position for first intercourse?

MARSHALL: The important thing about the best position for first intercourse is that it be comfortable both physically and psychologically to both man and woman. Only in this way can each give of himself or herself. If she is fearful of being squashed or hurt unduly in any way, she will not be able to relax; the muscles around the vagina will be tense, and the size of the opening will thereby be reduced. The fear or anxiety can be so great, usually due to unconscious factors, that the muscles go into involuntary spasm, and it is impossible to insert even a finger. If the muscles are relaxed, then the vaginal opening can perhaps be increased by spreading the legs far apart with the hips flexed (bent). Sometimes fear can be reduced by her being astride while the man is on his back, thereby giving her the active role and control of the insertion. There is too much made of the physical aspect of first intercourse.

PEG: Many young ladies who are still virgins go through extensive wedding preparations and strenuous parties prior to the wedding. When the wedding day comes, maybe the bride and groom have not had much sleep for several nights preceding it. They expect to hop into bed that first night and consummate their marriage, but are quite surprised that they have an unsatisfactory experience. Aside from fatigue, there is the couple's pattern of arousal. Couples who abstain from intercourse during their courtship may have spent three or four hours at a time petting. Once married, they expect to hop into bed and perform in ten minutes. Your arousal time is not changed that much by a wedding or civil-union ceremony. If you have taken a good long time snuggling and cuddling and smooching to get aroused before, then early in marriage you may still need a fair amount of time. I think some initial difficulty with intercourse arises from the woman not being adequately aroused before intercourse is attempted. Again, if the vagina is not adequately lubricated, it is an indication that she is not sufficiently aroused. It does not mean there is anything wrong with her; it just means that more time should be spent in foreplay.

Nudity

PEG: It may come as a surprise to some of you fellows, but some women are more concerned about their nudity than about the act of intercourse itself. Some inexperienced or minimally experienced women just cannot relax and give of themselves while nude. Of course, they should tell you so if they are aware of it. By the same token, a heavy flannel nightgown is not very stimulating to a man. Often a happy compromise will be a high quality satin-finish nightgown.

MARSHALL: So in summary, discomfort during initial intercourse will depend upon the thickness of the hymen, the size of its opening, and what stage of arousal is achieved prior to insertion of the penis. Arousal level will be affected by many factors: (1) preconceived ideas of the sex act; (2) ability to give of oneself totally and receive from the partner; (3) whether one partner or both are rested or fatigued; (4) whether the environment is free of potential distractions; (5) the appropriate quality and quantity of stimulation; and (6) whether or not maximally efficient contraception is mandatory, since pregnancies can and do result from first intercourse. Consequently, first intercourse should be deliberate and planned, including contraception. This deliberation does not contradict the need for spontaneity. The planning is before the love play; the spontaneity is during, just as one might plan a picnic, then act spontaneously during the picnic.

Chapter 5
Sex Before Long-term Commitment

Setting for Premarital Intercourse

MARSHALL: The circumstances and the environment in which most premarital or pre-relationship intercourse occurs are usually not nearly as secure as they should be. Often they are conducive to anything but a satisfying experience. One or both partners may be somewhat uneasy to begin with. Outside distractions, nervousness, pressure from a partner, needing to hurry, and unrealistic expectation may completely ruin the mood. The woman may not have an orgasm, which often leads to all sorts of misconceptions about herself and about sex from such an experience. The fellow may begin to wonder about himself, since he was not able to arouse or satisfy her. It is a lot less painful to attribute dissatisfaction to a physical reason than to a psychological reason or to the situation and circumstances. Hence, this idea of physical incompatibility enables him to say, "Too bad we didn't hit it off; we are both adequate sexually, just physically incompatible."

PEG: Regardless of what he said or how he said it, she may well conclude, "He doesn't want me anymore; I wasn't good enough for him." To answer these doubts, either the man or the woman or both may seek new partners, more so to reassure themselves of their sexual adequacy than to enjoy the relationship. Hence, they are understandably less able to give of themselves to their partner, and less likely to have a satisfying experience. This is particularly true if they choose a partner they are not particularly interested in as a person, and if they think more about their own performance during intercourse than they focus on their partner.

MARSHALL: The greatest distraction during intercourse is concern for one's own adequacy of performance. Once this concern supplants thoughts pertinent to stimulating one's partner and the partner's response to the stimulation, arousal levels drop, and the erection may be lost or vaginal lubrication resorbed. Either event will leave both partners scared as to "what's wrong with me?" and the cycle will be set to repeat itself.

Before we can consider what are the effects of sex outside of a committed relationship, we need to be aware of why each partner was engaging in it.

Reasons for Pre-relationship Intercourse

PEG: There are a number of reasons why people engage in intercourse without having established a long-term commitment. One is curiosity. Thus, one of the questions we often receive is: "Does curiosity pay?"

Curiosity

I think it depends on what you are curious about: the act in and of itself, in which case you may possibly be satisfied; or the act as an expression of a total, mutually open relationship with another person. In the latter case, the feelings you have for the particular person whose body you are sharing become quite important, and you may well be short-changed by pre-commitment or premarital sex. Intercourse for curiosity can also be costly if adequate thinking has not been done. Pregnancy may be the price. In addition, the individual who is just curious often finds a partner who has been quite active, and the cost may be venereal disease. There is a fair amount of initial intercourse going on among adolescents and young adults just for curiosity's sake.

Peer Pressure

Another reason for premarital intercourse may be peer pressure. Some adolescents are led to believe that the majority of their age-peers are having premarital intercourse and that, if they want to be like others, they should, too. Many who overstate the commonality of sexual behavior are strong individualists, yet somehow they do not want others to find "their thing." The main reason for this type of peer pressure is that an individual who is not sure of himself or of what he is doing can and frequently does take refuge in the belief that "everybody else is just like me." It is difficult for one person to murder another, but the lynch mob is somehow different. Also, "the thing to be done"—whether it is smoking, drinking, or making out—is always seen as big, brave, or adult. Young adolescents are often told by an older one that "you are not really grown up until you have had sex." People seldom realize that the demand to prove you are "as big as we are" is itself immature.

Sexual experience may also be sought in reaction to indirect peer pressure: "Gee, everybody else is doing it, and if I don't there must be something wrong with me. I sure don't want to let the guys (or the girls) think I'm inexperienced."

Inability to Set Limits

This feeling of inexperience has a broader social dimension, too. Some students get carried along because they do not know how to set a limit or terminate a date and still be on good terms. Many young people are subject to rules that are convenient for both sexes to hide behind, if they want to. Adolescents with less structure and supervision are required to be strong, self-confident individuals with their values and desires well thought out and their feelings under complete control. This includes a willingness to cite restrictions such as, "I have to be home by ten tonight," even if that is not actually true, in order to escape a situation with uncomfortable pressure. I think this is an unrealistic expectation for many. Thus pressure to be physically intimate, if not sexually active, is increased, often before the individuals or the relationship is ready for it. For some, this added pressure is enough to tip the scales of ambivalence toward intercourse. Intercourse under such circumstances is a predisposition to sexual difficulties.

In other individuals, the need to prove adequacy by acting big and sophisticated may have nothing to do with peers. The individual may need to feel that he or she is acceptable and attractive to a member of the opposite sex. The guy who is not quite sure that he is adequate as a man often feels he can "prove" it to himself by sexual activity, and gals can behave in the same way.

Proof of Sexual Adequacy

MARSHALL: I would like to add that the individuals who have the most concern about their own sexual adequacy are the ones who indeed have to be more active to reassure themselves constantly of their sexual adequacy, sexual attractiveness, and the security of their sexual identity. The Kinsey report confirmed that the lower the socio-economic class, the younger the age of individuals at first intercourse, and the more frequent the intercourse. This makes sense: If society has stripped an individual of many other ways to prove to himself he is a man, he will fall back on his biological manliness-sex. Likewise, many adolescent girls use sex to feel like a woman, even seeking to become mothers in order to feel grown up.

Can a person who doesn't have frequent or any premarital intercourse also be insecure? Doesn't your statement concerning this refer to those who have the opportunity for such activity?

PEG: Sure, I think it does. I do not mean to say that the only people who are active are those who are insecure. A lot of people enter each episode of sexual intercourse with some anxiety regarding their sexual adequacy at that particular time, but many inexperienced individuals feel insecure, of course.

MARSHALL: The answer is: certainly. You can be insecure and not engage in intercourse.

To Hold On to the Man

PEG: Absolutely. And I think another reason young women I have seen in my office are participating in intercourse is that they are afraid if they do not have intercourse with a fellow he is going to go with somebody who will. In essence, they are holding on to their boyfriend by means of intercourse. Adequate communication will be stymied right from the start. If you are just holding on to a fellow by having intercourse with him, you are not as likely to say that you are not quite ready yet or that you are not adequately aroused, because you might drive the guy toward some other gal. Similarly, those who feel inadequate sexually will be the last to say, "I am not ready yet."

But this is the sort of communication you need, particularly in early experience with intercourse. Much of sexual intercourse is innate behavior, but much must be learned. I think human sexual response is probably the most complicated psychological and physical intermeshing of mechanisms that has ever been investigated. It is tremendously complex; many things enter into it. Having sexual intercourse either with someone you are unable to communicate with because of any number of blocks, or with whom you do not have a sturdy enough relationship, steady enough and deep enough to allow for this type of communication, is really asking for trouble.

Initial intercourse is going to leave an impression, and as you know first impressions are important. They may be entirely wrong, but they are hard to reverse. If initially you engage in intercourse in a compromising situation and in a relationship that is less than ideal, you will have an experience that is far less than ideal. Having nothing to compare it to, you may consider it the norm: a price to premarital sex besides the pregnancy risk.

Expression of Anger

MARSHALL: Another reason people engage in premarital sex, and fortunately a rather rare one, is as an expression of anger; e.g., to get back at their parents or an ex-sweetheart. This, of course, involves the other party's finding out about the affair. Both men and women may act this way, and sometimes with women it may also involve pregnancy.

PEG: I have seen many young ladies with this motivation for intercourse. One came into my office and asked for contraceptives because she said she had been quite active sexually, having intercourse three or four times a week for about two-and-a-half months. A pelvic exam substantiated her statement of sexual activity. I asked what contraceptives she had been using. She looked blank, hesitated, and then said none.

> "And why then after two-and-a-half months do you want the pill?"
>
> "I don't know. I knew I was taking a chance all along, but now it doesn't seem worth it."
>
> "Worth what?"
>
> "Well, when I first came to school, I was failing in my work to get at my folks; then I realized it was hurting me more than them, so I stopped."
>
> "And started taking a chance on getting pregnant? How would your folks react to that?"
>
> "Yeah, I see what you mean."
>
> "Why not just tell 'em off about whatever you are mad about? It's a lot more satisfying, and sometimes even parents

change when the issue is clearly stated with some depth of feeling."

Just Pleasure

What do you say about a sexual relationship where neither party is considering the process of marriage, where both parties are perfectly aware of the other's stance and are engaging in the relationship strictly for pleasure?

PEG: A common reason among men for premarital intercourse is "just pleasure." Neither of us has ever seen a young woman who gave this as the only reason, or with whom we thought this was the only reason. The women these fellows have as partners have another reason; hence, this question is not a relevant one from our experience.

MARSHALL: To have an affair where the relationship is strictly mutual pleasure, where you do not care for the other person as a personality, is to delude yourself as to what sex can be all about, and to greatly lower or modify the expectations that you might have of a sexual partner later. Do you really care about the other individual's pleasure, or are you just using somebody else's body to masturbate with? Granted, it is more pleasurable than using your hand. In terms of your relationship to her, it is prostitution without money. We need to take only one step further, and we have the feeling behind the expression "Screw you," namely: "I hope somebody uses you intimately for their own pleasure without any other consideration of you."

Civilization takes a great step forward when it does away with parentally arranged marriages, because it is not love, because people's individual personalities matter. I grant marriage is more than sex, much more; but when you say sex only for pleasure, are you not saying that in sex the individual's personality does not really matter?

If, on the other hand, you cannot consider a lasting relationship for some reason (be it incompatibility of religion, your school and career plans, or something else that you both hold important), and if there is a genuine, mutual feeling of respect and giving of your whole selves to each other, then I think it is quite a different matter.

PEG: Some young women just feel it is part of being liberal.

MARSHALL: This fits in with a few who apparently feel their fathers want or expect them to be active sexually. These fathers tend to be very permissive about their daughters' behaviors. But if, either inadvertently or via her pregnancy, one of these fathers finds out his daughter is sexually active, he will be hurt or angry. The depth of hurt these young ladies experience and the feeling of betrayal is quite deep.

To Give Unselfishly of Self

PEG: Young ladies sometimes engage in premarital intercourse with the feeling that for the first time they are able to do something for somebody else, to give of themselves, to make the young man happy. Many come from families that are moderately well-to-do, and they have not been required to work or to make a contribution to anyone else. Doing well in school has been their primary job, and they feel this is kind of selfish. Some guy says, "You can really do something for me. You can make me happy; you can give me enjoyment." It is quite ego inflating. Or the gal may just have a need to give, and this is the way she has found to do it. It may not make a great deal of difference who the fellow is. And he may feel the arrangement is for mutual pleasure. In a sense it is, but her pleasure is not the pure pleasure of hedonism; it is her needing to prove to herself that she is worth something to someone.

Carried Away by Emotions

MARSHALL: Sometimes people get involved in premarital intercourse simply because they are carried away by their feelings. Too often the young ladies who act on their feelings without thinking, who do not plan, get pregnant and show up in a doctor's office, not really understanding how it all happened. As a boy grows up, he sees suggestive images and may get aroused sexually. He gets experience controlling sexual feelings in small doses. But with the need for atmosphere and a whole mood, there is not as much opportunity for girls to become sexually aroused in small doses as they grow up. Frequently, these feelings are so strong the first time the adolescent girl really experiences them, that she does not know how to handle them. One of the signs of maturity is the ability to control the expression of feelings while mindful of others. The expression of strong feelings of sexual excitement no more needs to culminate in intercourse than strong anger needs to culminate in punching somebody in the nose. In fact, intercourse may be an entirely inappropriate expression of feelings of sexual arousal; in essence, a sexual tantrum.

Is heavy petting advisable as a preparation or practice so you are more aware of your sexual pattern?

PEG: Usually, just as Marshall has said, it allows both sexes to experience sexual feelings in degrees and to gain experience with these feelings. It is also enjoyable in its own right. But it is not a prerequisite. I think the most important thing is that you have decided in your own mind how you are going to act and where you are going to draw the line as to how far you want to go in petting.

Expression of Intimacy

MARSHALL: Young adults are struggling with the problem of how to be intimate. Many engage in premarital sexual intercourse just in an attempt to be intimate. Intimacy with another person has both psychological and physical components, and sexual intercourse should include the heights of both. Psychological intimacy has more to do with the sharing of hopes, fears, aspirations, and disappointments; of exposing a little of your felt weakness, than it does with a sharing of bodies. The act of intercourse, to be sure, is the height of physical intimacy, but that need not involve psychological intimacy. Consider the prostitute. In the act of intercourse there needs to be a total intimacy between the total selves of the individuals involved. Intimacy means knowing the other's individual personality in depth, knowing his or her needs; knowing him or her so well as to know there is not another similar person in all the world. Intimacy does not occur just between men and women. It can and does occur between two women, or two men, and sometimes a group.

Expression of Love

The last reason we want to mention, by far the most frequent one given by young women and rather frequent with the fellows, too, is premarital intercourse as an expression of love. People in love usually desire a long-term committed relationship, usually leading to marriage. There are many factors to consider before deciding that sex is an appropriate expression of love before a relationship based on more than new feelings has been established.

Effects on Married Life

Could premarital sex in any way affect my married life?

MARSHALL: There are some for whom I am sure the answer would be yes, and there are others for whom the answer would be no. If you can give as an individual, give of your total self psychologically and physically, including thoughts, feelings, and actions; if your partner can give to you in the same way; if you are both free to receive from the other as an individual; and if you both can acknowledge the other's giving (and have given adequate thought to preventing pregnancy and disease transmission), then I do not think it is going to have any detrimental effect on your married life.

That is not quite as simple as it sounds. Giving of your total self includes giving of your superego or conscience, too. It means an intimate relationship. It means meeting the needs of the other, a place of comfort and of proper atmosphere. It means opening up and taking the other in, into yourself. If, on the other hand, you can only half-heartedly give of yourself, or if your partner can only half-heartedly give to you, then I think your first experience in sex is going to be much different than what sex is meant to be. First impressions are first impressions. It takes effort; it takes re-concentration and reconsideration to correct them.

Then there is the whole concept of so-called physical incompatibility we talked about, which points up the other very important element in premarital sexual activity, or any sexual activity: the need for an ongoing relationship. You need to be able to grow and develop in a sexual relationship as with any other kind of relationship. When you start having intercourse, it is like learning to walk or ride a bicycle: you stumble and fall sometimes. You need to be able to communicate to your partner that the stimulation of one part of your body was a little rough; or that this was the part you liked most; or that was the part you would like to do a little further. You need somebody with whom you feel close enough and secure enough to be able to communicate these things during the act, or the next day, or the day after that, and still be able to pick up the relationship and carry it forward from there. Nonverbal communication is best, but by all means use words if you need to. No doubt this is an individual thing and will vary a great deal with your own sense of values and the sense of values of your partner, and with your perception of each other's sense of values. If you feel that your lover is completely giving, it is quite different from feeling that you have in any way tricked or set up or taken advantage of him or her. Those are the contingencies that you have to be able to answer in a particular circumstance to be able to decide what effect premarital sex will have on a later relationship.

PEG: Pregnancy or sexually transmitted disease (STD) would certainly have an effect!

Effects on Love

How do you think having sexual relations with somebody you don't love or particularly care about would affect your relationship with somebody you do love? Specifically, say that you're away in college and love someone at home. If you have intercourse with someone in school whom you don't particularly care about, might it not take some of the beauty and feeling of sacredness out of what you do with the person whom you do love?

MARSHALL: I think the answer is yes, and I think the question has actually said it better than I could. Very likely, this situation involves using the body of someone you do not care about at all as a kind of fantasy representation of the one you love. When a person is really in love, it may be difficult to have a successful masturbatory fantasy; therefore, the incidence of masturbation goes down sharply. The same holds true for intercourse. If you need a fantasy all the time, every time, then your actual relationship is not satisfying. However, the converse is not necessarily true; absence of a sexual fantasy during intercourse does not necessarily indicate an adequate love relationship.

Is it an expression of love or is it just sexual maneuver for physical gratification? If intercourse is not love, then how are the two of you using it? Do you really find it worthwhile?

To Make Love Complete

Does premarital sex increase or complete the love between a couple?

PEG: Sex is the height of physical intimacy. The act of intercourse should complete or fulfill the expression of love between a couple. But there is no pat answer to that question because the premarital part may have the opposite effect on given individuals. Commitment such as marriage completes intimacy.

Marriage

MARSHALL: Let us take up the effects of premarital intercourse and marriage. Marriage is a legal act. But aside from that, and more important to the success of the union, there is a psychological commitment that goes with the legal act. The psychological aspect of marriage is a personal commitment of one partner to the other to strive for happiness and the attainment of a "oneness." We have tried to say that to have a successful premarital experience, a couple must come quite close to achieving the psychological aspects of marriage without the legal aspects. You need a trusting relationship; you need the right atmosphere; you need the other person to give to you without feeling that somebody is going to do something wrong; you need to be free of fear of being abandoned. I think that if the two partners feel this way, why not get married? If you are not willing to make that commitment, then what kind of "love" is it?

Aside from the legal aspect, the difference between marriage and the thrust of some of these questions—that is, premarital sex with love, and commitment, and fulfillment, etc.—is the time aspect. Does your love commitment to each other extend past the one-nighter? Is your love commitment to each other for a week, a month, a year? Or is it a total commitment forever? How long do you expect this love to last? If your love is not a total, enveloping love, a love that psychologically drives you to possess and possess forever, then it is not what it might be. It is one thing to whisper it in the ear; it is quite another to say it publicly. The difference has to do with how much you really mean it.

Partner's History

What does it mean to a man if his girlfriend has had premarital intercourse with somebody else?

MARSHALL I think this is entirely a personal thing and depends on his values. It can hurt terribly. Some may be just a little hurt or disappointed. To others (most), it makes minimal difference. The opposite is also true: your feelings about whether or not the man you marry has already had intercourse depends on your values.

Can your husband tell if you have had intercourse?

PEG: He usually can if he is a doctor. It requires a rather specific examination which I doubt most husbands would do before they have intercourse with their wives. Though detection is possible with a medically sophisticated individual, the likelihood is that he cannot, and that he would not even if he could. (See our discussion of the hymen.)

Considerations Prior to Premarital Intercourse

What is sort of the minimum a person should consider before she has premarital intercourse?

MARSHALL: First, you should consider the relationship. Is it to be an expression of love? If so, what are you calling love? If not, what is the rationale? Second, you should consider whether or not you are living up to the dictates of your own value system. I think basically that you should be able to give of yourself in feeling, thinking, and acting. I think you should have an ongoing and steady, trusting relationship. Trust should be of such proportions that freedom to communicate would exist after the act as well as during the act. It should take place in a setting where both can feel rather relaxed, unhurried, and comfortable. Psychologically, whether or not people can give of themselves depends on their own value system, as well as on the person they are giving to. I really do not think that one partner needs to be experienced. This often causes many more problems than it avoids. Third, but not less important, an adequate method of contraception is needed, which usually means either the pill or the combination of intravaginal foam and a condom.

"Backing Up"

You were talking about a couple who had been going together for a while and they had gone quite far, but wanted to set a limit that was not quite as far as they had already gone. Could they do that?

MARSHALL: Yes. It is much more difficult to "back up" than to set a limit in advance and hold it, but it is done.

PEG: If you find that you both do not want intercourse before you are married, but that you are getting more and more aroused when you are alone together, you could double date. Do not get into situations where you are too tempted. Do not be alone where one of you lives. Many couples, when they find that they get too aroused if they are alone together, just avoid that situation.

MARSHALL: I do not think you really have to go quite that far. I think you can set a limit, and if you have good control over the expression of your feelings, you can hold to it. You can become more intimate without being physically intimate. This certainly might include very heavy petting or mutual masturbation. Again, I think where the two of you draw the line depends on your own value systems.

You should expect enough respect of your values and have a strong enough relationship to say, "We have been petting and we are really going a little further than I feel comfortable going. I would like to stop at point X." You should be able to say that, ask how your partner feels about it, discuss it openly, and arrive at a mutual decision. If your partner loves you and wants to make you happy, if he or she cares as much about your happiness as his or her own, then he or she deserves to know when you feel pushed beyond the point of comfort. In a love relationship you actually should feel obligated to speak out. Your partner has a right to know. This applies to all areas of married life, not just sex.

Self-control

PEG: I strongly feel that the ability and willingness to control the expression of one's feelings is a part of maturation. This is a part of growing up, of being mature. You are not accountable for your feelings; that is, for the fact that you feel sexually excited. You cannot wish them away. You cannot say, "I'm not going to feel aroused." But you can modify the situation and thereby your feelings. You are entirely accountable for how you act on the basis of these feelings. It is easy to see the difference between children and adults in this respect. When a baby wants something, he wants it right then. He wails, he hollers; and the only way to make him stop is to satisfy his craving for whatever it is. Part of maturing is the ability to put off the fulfillment of feelings to a later date when they are more appropriate. And this holds true for sexual desires as well as others. The immature person feels that he has to have intercourse every time he is aroused. This is just as immature as hauling off and hitting somebody every time you are angry. There is a time and a place. As Pete Seeger has popularized Ecclesiastes in the song "Turn, Turn, Turn," there is a time for everything under heaven: a time for war and a time for peace; a time to weep and a time to laugh; a time to embrace, and a time to refrain from embracing.

Chapter 6
Ambivalence and the Sex Act

MARSHALL: At times, individuals have mixed or mutually contradictory feelings simultaneously. This is called ambivalence. Frigidity, impotence, and premature ejaculation may result from ambivalent feelings. Frigidity is the term applied to the aversion women feel due to experiencing pain with intercourse, or because they cannot respond to sexual stimulation. Impotence in the male is the inability to obtain or maintain an erection sufficient for intercourse. Premature ejaculation in the male occurs just before, during, or shortly after insertion of the penis into the vagina. Generally speaking, frigidity or impotence is the result of an individual's inability to give wholly of himself or to receive from the other person.

Frigidity

Can a woman be just a little bit frigid?

PEG: There are various gradations of frigidity. The most severe grade would be sexual intercourse that is painful. The next grade would be a feeling of unpleasantness. Another form of frigidity would be when the act is considered not particularly pleasurable but not uncomfortable either, just something to go along with. In the least severe gradation, intercourse is pleasurable, but orgasm is not reached.

Frigid or Clumsy

Is there anything to the saying "There is no such thing as a frigid woman, just a clumsy man?"

PEG: Perhaps in some cases, but clumsy men need not be so. It is the woman's responsibility to communicate what she desires for sexual stimulation. Men do not have divine guidance, nor do they inherently know what to do to arouse a particular woman; she must feel free to communicate her desires on a moment-to-moment basis. Frequently a woman will not know what she wants until she realizes she is not getting it. A caress that is exquisitely pleasurable on one occasion may cause indifference or even feel unpleasant at a subsequent time, and vice versa. Sexual arousal is not a push-button occurrence.

Lack of Sex Instruction

My parents never instructed me in sex. It was never discussed in our home except for, "Don't get pregnant before marrying or you'll be disowned." I find myself afraid of sex because of this and have an actual fear of getting pregnant. What can I do?

Now this kind of feeling has nothing to do with clumsy men, and the person should seek individual counseling. There is another question implied here, which asks, How do you teach a child about sex? Children's underlying attitudes toward sex are formed from what they sense of their parents' attitudes, which may also include the emotional tone a parent uses when answering questions about sex. The comfortableness a parent has in answering the questions is more important than the information. Misconceptions of knowledge are fairly easily corrected; misconceived attitudes are not so easy to change. Basically, if a child can formulate a question, he is old enough for a simple answer. Do not take the one or two questions as invitations for a long, drawn-out sex talk. Keep it brief. The sit-down sex talk is unnatural, especially for children. It is preferable to talk while the child is doing something with you, such as making cookies or fixing the lawnmower. There are some simple ways to tell children the facts of life, and some good books are available for anyone to consult.

It has always struck me as odd that parents have so much difficulty telling their children about sex, something that is rational and about which they know something. Yet somehow they have no difficulty explaining war, or killing. Why?

Sex Without Orgasm

What's wrong if a woman appears more than willing to go to bed, yet she doesn't have orgasm, or, as you described, increased tension. Is she frigid?

PEG: There are probably unconscious factors, ambivalent feelings, that prevent her from giving of her total self. This might be frigidity. Frigidity occurs in varying degrees, from the inability of a woman to relax pelvic muscles enough so that intercourse becomes actually painful, to the situation you described. Sex, for too many, is considered dirty, taboo, and not talked about; or at least too embarrassing to discuss. That is one of the reasons so many people and even older people with experience have so many unanswered questions about sex. Many of us were not really "talked to" about sex by our parents. This attitude cannot be wholly put aside when someone says to himself or herself, "I am married now and will change my attitude." Feelings are facts. Sexual response is probably the most complex reaction that goes on in anybody, particularly in women. Why this woman is permissive and raises no objections to the act, yet is apparently unable to enjoy it—or at least unable to be adequately stimulated—goes back to her thoughts and feelings. She may be unsure of you as a person or of how gentle you will be. There may not have been adequate foreplay before insertion of the penis, or she may have scruples she is not even admitting to herself. As Marshall said before, women are very easily distracted. Any sort of thought or external disturbance can completely lower her from any plateau of sexual excitement. It is just tremendously complex. Perhaps her difficulty may have something to do with her partner or with thoughts about her parents. This is why we say that if you are going to have intercourse as an expression of love, you have got to have a real relationship going which has honest and open communication so that you can ask: Was there need for more stimulation? Was there anything that I could have done, or should have done, or should not have done?

There may have been a communication problem. Possibly the woman thought that if she represented her need it might be taken as a put-down since men are "supposed to know" how to stimulate women.

Do you think that since she didn't have a climax on that one occasion, that it's fair to say she wouldn't on the next, or do you think it might be different?

PEG: That depends entirely on what the reason was.

MARSHALL: There are many, many reasons why the woman may not have an orgasm and the man does. Even in a happily adjusted married couple, the woman may not have orgasm every time. I do not know that it basically has anything to do with technique. To the extent that it does, if you are free to talk to each other about it, I do not see any reason to call it quits. If you are going to call it quits over something like that, you really ought to look at what you are calling love.

I would never say it was love.

MARSHALL: All right, that may be the whole thing. If the woman suspects she is not loved, then it stands to reason that she is not going to be totally able to give of herself. People need to feel loved, totally loved, and totally cared for. What was her reason for wanting intercourse with you? Did she love you? Or did she only care about you as a penis-possessing person and not as an individual? Was she out to prove her sexual adequacy?

Before you give up and seek a different partner, think what her response will be. "I wasn't good enough for him; he doesn't want me again; I'm inadequate sexually." And with more doubts she goes out to prove she is adequate; then the next time, she is so concerned watching her own reactions that she cannot give. Consequently, she does not get as aroused as she did with you and gets dumped again, and the cycle is set to repeat itself.

Love Without Sex

Where can a girl who is frigid find somebody to marry her without sex?

MARSHALL: I think it would be more important that you get some consultation regarding what you are calling frigidity and find out what your psychological make-up is and what sort of blocks you have on this problem.

PEG: Again, I think this involves the problem of women thinking they are frigid when really their sexual attempts have been under such compromising circumstances that they are just unable to respond or relax at all. This is one of the prices of sexual experimentation in a relationship where there is no true commitment to each other. For example, a woman is at her boyfriend's apartment and his roommate is due back any minute. Nevertheless, they pop into the bedroom anyway, and she cannot perform. It is not surprising at all. She thinks she is frigid, or they call it "physical incompatibility." Again, female sexual arousal patterns are very complex, and a woman needs to feel completely secure with the fellow. Many cannot relax during sexual intimacy without commitment, possibly even the commitment of marriage.

MARSHALL: I do not think any minimally experienced woman should consider herself frigid at this stage, especially when there are unsatisfactory experiences as a possible basis. If that is your rationale, then delay your conclusions until you do have a trusting love relationship with something of a permanent commitment, and then freely communicate your feelings. All couples should work on enhancing each other's sexual gratification. Each has to learn the sexual responses of the other and very likely of themselves, too. On the other hand, if you feel you are—or are likely to be—frigid because of your attitudes, the attitudes you got from your parents, and because of your feeling that sex is dirty, then wait until you are in love. There is something about intimacy and being in love that calls for physical expression. As this urge for physical expression increases in petting, you will become aroused; you will have a greater pelvic awareness and will somehow want to use it in some vague way in the physical expression of that intimacy. Often it is not dirty anymore; it is just part of you and part of him and all of each of you belonging together.

Many women who have not experienced feelings of intimacy with men, or many feelings of sexual arousal, feel that sex is dirty. They may have some catching up to do. They could benefit from a prolonged courtship and from a lot of so-called heavy petting. If you are afraid you may be frigid, you can tell your partner in advance. But I would not consider her dishonest if she did not mention her fear, unless she had been happily committed to another previously and in that relationship concluded she was frigid. If you are in love, but afraid you are frigid, talk over your feelings with someone who can help you. Pick someone you respect and who has experience counseling people, someone whom you think would be knowledgeable about sexual matters. These attributes are much more important than his or her profession. Physicians, social workers, clergymen, psychologists, and psychiatrists should be considered. A woman who is frigid because of attitudes formed in childhood may need psychiatric treatment.

There definitely are people for whom sexual activity is unimportant or even a negative matter. Reportedly, sexless marriages are more common than is generally realized. There are people for whom a sexless marriage is a way of life. Such a union can be as comfortable and as rewarding as are any of the more conventional relationships for other people.

Penis Size and Frigidity

Is the size of the male organ directly related to the effectiveness of the male sex act?

MARSHALL: Masters and Johnson answered that pretty thoroughly, and the answer is no. In their study, they found that a large penis in the flaccid state does not enlarge proportionately as much during erection as the smaller penis. Although there may be significant differences in penis sizes when they are in the relaxed state, the maximum difference in the size when erect is only about an inch. But more importantly, it is from the first third of the vagina and from the clitoris that a woman gets her stimulation, and no erect penises were observed to be less than about three times that length. Hence, effective stimulation is not related to the length of the penis or the depth of penetration.

Physical Incompatibility of Genitalia

Is there such a problem as the male organ being too big and the female organ being too small in sexual relations?

PEG: The answer is no; that is, aside from the intact hymen condition, which would prevent the admission of any size penis. (See Chapter 4.) The vagina is a very expandable organ with many folds of tissue in its walls. As the vagina expands, the size of these folds decreases. It takes something the size of a baby's head at birth to really stretch the vagina. (By the way, the pains of labor are primarily from contractions of the uterus, not from the stretching of the vagina.) In a state of excitation—that is, if the woman is stimulated adequately—the vagina dilates considerably even prior to the insertion of the penis. As stimulation and excitement continue into the plateau stage, the outer third of the vagina becomes engorged, narrowing the vaginal outlet. A woman may also be so tense as a result of varying psychological factors that the muscles around the outlet of the vagina go into an involuntary spasm to the extent that insertion of the penis is impossible. This state is completely involuntary on her part; she has no control over it.

Communication and Relationship

Then is there a technical definition of sexual incompatibility, or is it just that one of the partners doesn't really enjoy it?

MARSHALL: Incompatibility is apparently a bothersome problem. It is a psychological thing. If it is sexual technique, then it is communication failure of technique. If it is not technique, then look to the relationship. What is each of you trying to get out of the relationship? If each of you has different aims and goals for your relationship, you would do well to see just how they differ. For example, one may want pleasure, the other love. Evaluate this difference and what it means to each of you; then decide whether or not to continue the relationship.

Where the goals are the same, I have never seen a sex problem in which the basic difficulty was not a matter of communication. It is not always a lack of communication about sex, but since sex is an expression of intimacy, it usually gets involved secondarily, if not primarily. Basically, the problem is a feeling of being slighted, of being unloved, or of not being given proper consideration. If this feeling is not expressed, the resentment slips out or is delivered intentionally at the first "justifiable" opportunity. Yet, the original slight is never mentioned, and as feelings build up, sex naturally gets involved.

Importance of Anger

Anger does have a place because it communicates how much something is disliked. This information is just as essential for people in love as what it is that is disliked. The degrees of liking and loving are obvious. The depth of love is communicated rather readily in our culture, but somehow we do not acknowledge the same need to communicate the depth of our dislike. Watch how you communicate your anger, but be sure to communicate it.

Premature Ejaculation

What about premature ejaculation?

Masters and Johnson report a 97 percent cure rate when treating this condition of premature ejaculation, which is far superior to any other approach. They found the premature ejaculator had a history of intercourse which was practically devoid of consideration for the female's sexual tensions, and that often there was a premium on speed. For example, intercourse performed when there is a fear of momentary discovery or in houses of prostitution can place a premium on speed. Usually a couple has tried to cope with the problem of rapid ejaculation by reducing the stimulation the female gives the male, and by having the male distract himself mentally by such maneuvers as thinking about something unrelated to sex or biting his lip. This is not helpful and will usually lead to secondary impotence. However, Masters and Johnson discovered a physiologic reflex that will delay the ejaculation. The female partner incorporates this reflex repeatedly in the love play. They also make sure she communicates that she wants and enjoys her partner's sexual responses. In this way the premature ejaculator reprograms or reconditions himself to adequate sexual functioning.

Delayed Ejaculation

How long can ejaculation be delayed once the penis is in the vagina? Is it harmful to try to delay orgasm as long as possible?

MARSHALL: Ejaculation can be delayed for an extended period of time, even measured in hours. At times, some couples, after the male inserts his penis, just go to sleep when they feel close, but do not feel really exuberant. Needless to say, this is a couple who are quite comfortable with themselves and each other. (Factors affecting the "Duration of Intercourse" are discussed in Chapter 2.) A man may partially train himself to delay his ejaculation by knowing his sexual responses and practice. It is in no way harmful to delay ejaculation. The only reasons for doing so are for enjoyment of variations and to enable the woman to achieve one or several orgasms.

PEG: Certainly there is no need for a woman to attempt to delay orgasm, since she is capable of a multi-orgasmic response.

Impotence

What about loss of erection before ejaculation?

The inability to obtain or maintain an erection is called impotence. Unlike premature ejaculation, impotence is primarily psychological. The mores of many societies have put essentially all responsibility for the sexual functioning of a couple on the male. Innately, or by divine guidance, men are supposed to know how to perform for themselves and bring satisfaction and pleasure to their partners. The female's contribution in some couples is simple availability. Distraction is the basic cause of secondary impotence, and the foremost distraction is fear of performance. Once genuine doubt as to performance has arisen, a man is apt to be so distracted by "observing" his sexual performance that he cannot perform. Of course, other thoughts and feelings may be so distracting that they interfere with giving or receiving to the point of impotence. There are numerous examples of such failures, most of which are the result of the man's lack of full recognition of his own value system. For example, a man may perceive that the woman is scared to death, but tells himself it does not matter to him, she is plenty willing. If he is correct that it does not make any difference to him, then he will have no difficulty; but, if it does make a difference to him, he may be impotent. Another man may find himself distracted by continuing thoughts that the woman is married, although he believed such thoughts would not make any difference to him. Do not get upset if you lose erection under such circumstances until you have learned something more about your value system. Either your value system or your action will need to change to be harmonious. Masters and Johnson deal with the problem of secondary impotence by assuring both the man and the woman that the sexual function is a natural process. Their approach is to help them clear away the distractions and help them concentrate on each other rather than on themselves. They report about 70 percent success with the condition of secondary impotence.

Chapter 7
Incompatibility:
Physical and Psychological

Size of the Vagina

How big is the vagina?

I think the questions actually implied here are: How big is the penis? How big does it get when excited? How big is the vagina? Are couples sometimes incompatible because of size difference?

PEG: The vagina is an expansible organ; it can expand enough for the delivery of a baby. Therefore, there really is no problem about whether a penis will be too large to be accommodated in the vagina. Basically, there is no true physical incompatibility, especially after the hymen has been enlarged, which occurs at first intercourse. The vagina is more a potential than a real space. In an unaroused state its walls are collapsed together; with arousal it lubricates and expands.

Size of the Penis

MARSHALL: The size of the penis will vary with how cold it is outside and with the state of excitement. I do not think most women are concerned about the size of the non-erect penis. Actually, the size of the penis is relatively unimportant in regard to effective sexual functioning since the vagina has nerve endings only in the outer third. Thus, all penises are big enough to satisfy both partners.

Psychological Incompatibility

MARSHALL: Incompatibility is basically psychological. There are many feelings that prevent the woman, the man, or both from sharing themselves with each other. To be able to give freely of one's total self, and to be able to receive from the other in all aspects, these involve an openness to the other, a giving and receiving of feeling, thought, and action. Hopefully, the basic feeling is love.

Giving freely of one's thoughts in this context means communicating those little (or big) feelings or the thoughts that might detract from the fullest, richest giving. For example, a woman who can give freely may be distracted by the thought and fear that she might be squashed by her partner's weight. When she communicates this fear to her partner, he can usually reassure her so that she is able to give more of her total self.

Receiving the other person's thoughts means being sensitive and considerate of each other's ideas and feelings, even if they seem foolish and are illogical. For example, a woman who is at ease having intercourse may not be at ease if she is nude because she feels her nudity is "an invasion of her privacy" while somehow a penis in her vagina is not. Never make fun of such feelings. They are part of your partner. You may question them and discuss them, but you need to respect his or her right to them, and treat them with a loving consideration. Receiving is as important as giving.

And there are acts that go together to make up the physical acts; each person must not only be able to give and receive stimulation in the sexual areas, but to give and receive with the face and eyes as well. This mutual giving and receiving of one's total self, one's being, makes sex what it can be. Anything else is much less. Can you give of yourself as a whole, as an individual whole? Can you give all parts of yourself to him or her? Can you accept him or her as an individual, or are you psychologically dividing up the other person and accepting only the sex organs? Do not think that the experience you get with a "quick make" is all that there is to sex. Basically physical incompatibility usually occurs because of distractions. For women the most common distractions are those which disrupt the mood or atmosphere. Even in married life a baby's cry, a dripping faucet, or car headlights passing through the room may puncture the atmosphere for a woman and drop her from any plateau of sexual arousal. She can also be distracted by concern over their privacy being invaded or a fear of pain or pregnancy. For men, on the other hand, the most common distractions are their own thoughts, especially concerning their sexual performance. They may become more of an observer than a performer and hence lose ability to perform. Men are less subject to environmental distractions than women. The truism of this statement is reflected in the exaggeration that it takes a shotgun in the back to distract a man.

One couple I saw had been married for about a year. Initially, sexual intercourse had been very satisfying, but for the past six months the wife had had great difficulty becoming aroused. She had begun to fear that she was frigid, and her husband was quite concerned, too. In discussing their problem, the only significant difference in the past six months we found was that they had moved from their apartment to the one which was directly above it. While they had lived in the first apartment, they had frequently heard the bed creaking above them and had chuckled about it. After moving upstairs, the wife was completely distracted by the thought of other people in adjacent apartments being aware of their sexual activity and chuckling at them. A new set of bedsprings cured her "frigidity."

Chapter 8
Intimacy Without Intercourse

When a couple has been dating for a long time, say over a year, is it natural for their sexual activities to become more intimate? Is it possible to avoid this?

Growth of a Relationship

MARSHALL: It is natural for the relationship to become more intimate. Psychologically, as we have said, there is a sharing of deep feelings, exposure of self-felt weaknesses, and dreaming and planning together. The physical side will naturally become more intimate, too. There are physical intimacies that create strong feelings of closeness that are not genitally arousing; a soft touch of the fingertips to the lips; a deft, gentle stroke across the side of the neck. Watch movies and you will see many examples of deeply expressed intimacy that do not necessarily progress to intercourse.

Mutually seductive physical acts also tend to increase. Slow progress may have advantages: if you do not get to breast play in the first month or so, you have more room in which to increase physical intimacy short of intercourse. The same may be said of fingering. But be careful here! Many people take fingering to be only a few minutes from intercourse. You will do well to know how your partner will interpret allowing these intimacies.

Transcultural Misunderstanding

PEG: A coed who had been raped had several bruises on her thighs and other signs of a forceful penetration, and she was afraid she was pregnant. But she did not call it rape; she called it a transcultural misunderstanding.

MARSHALL: This is an important point. Physical intimacies are interpreted differently in different cultures, sometimes quite differently. Where there are obvious cultural differences, both parties are on guard against misunderstandings. However, more commonly, transcultural misunderstandings occur between people of ostensibly similar cultures. In World War II, the soldiers had more communication difficulties of this type with British women than they did with women of any other nationality. Even in this country, many different interpretations may be attributed to the same sexual behavior. Usually they follow socio-economic, racial, and sectional differences. Do not be misunderstood.

Sexual Reputations

PEG: Reputations can cause trouble, too. Reputations may be built on empty boasts. When some students start a new school, or when anyone moves to a new community, they try to create an identity of being sexually in the know. They may be overreacting to peer pressure. They boast; they strut; but often they do not actually have intercourse. People who talk big about anything are often the non-doers. Then somebody dates him or her strictly for sex, solely on reputation. When turned down, he or she wonders, "What's wrong with me?" There is resentment and a questioning of his or her own sexual attractiveness and adequacy, which may occur during the date itself. For example, the man with the big sexual reputation may not be very aggressive early enough, so the woman questions her sexual adequacy and tries to provoke the sexual attraction she had expected to fend off. He then perceives that she is asking for it, and if she really was not, there is a problem.

Regardless of what transpires during the evening, the disappointed person is not likely to tell his or her buddies that the person with the big sexy reputation did not make out. The cycle is set to repeat itself.

Once a reputation like this gets established, it is very, very difficult to change. (In fact, with everybody you date pushing you, you may come to believe that the whole community is one big orgy.) I once saw a college coed in the office who was asked to leave her sorority for what was termed gross sexual promiscuity, but the pelvic exam revealed that she was a virgin.

Turning On

How can you keep from turning on a man?

PEG: I think that this is a very serious and legitimate question. Many men suppose that you expect them to be turned on, so they are really complimenting you in letting you know that you have turned them on. Would you really want to go with a fellow for several dates who was not stimulated by you? After one of our college talks on sex, a young woman came up to us afterwards and said, "I've been out with this guy four times; he's never made any advances. How can I tell whether he is a perfect gentleman or a homosexual?" Many men think that you expect to be pushed, and they also believe that you will set your own limits. Many of them will be relieved when you do.

MARSHALL: The question is not really how you keep from turning them on, but how you regulate the heat. Basically, I think you have to decide at some moment away from the man how far you are willing to go. Then, hold that limit consistently. The key is consistency. Once a man knows the limit, and once he has tested it and sees you mean it, he will not push you beyond it if he respects you and cares about you. But, if your limit varies from date to date, he will have to push and test each time. Set your limit and hold it, and he will respect it and you.

PEG: Some men tell me that they have had intercourse with every woman they have gone with since they were eighteen (which may be years), except the one they are going to marry. As one of them said, "It's not that I don't want it; it's just that she can't do it. It means that much to her." This situation is not uncommon.

Setting Limits

How will the man be affected by the woman setting the limits? How will he react?

MARSHALL: I do not think it will frustrate him unless you have led him to believe, perhaps in some small way, that you are willing to have intercourse. Oh, many will probably push, and will act frustrated, but will not be psychologically frustrated or resentful. This is why you need to set a consistent limit to establish his expectation level. I guess anything short of complete intercourse is physically frustrating to some extent. However, if you also show your attitude (the attitude is more important than the words) or say, "I like you (or love you), I care about you, but nevertheless this is the limit that I am setting, this is my value system," I would expect that he could take his physical frustration in stride. If he cannot control the expression of his emotions or have this much respect for you and your value system, he is not a very mature person.

Petting Without Intercourse

Is sexual arousal which does not terminate in intercourse physically or mentally harmful for the male or female?

PEG: There are many couples who pet heavily but postpone intercourse. In the female, this may result in pelvic aching and cramps similar to menstrual cramps. The discomfort begins shortly after petting stops and may last up to half an hour. In the man, there is similar pain in the testes, beginning about the same time period. The pain is due to distensions of the tissues with blood and other fluids. There is no other harmful effect, only the discomfort.

Orgasm Without Intercourse

Is it possible to cause a girl to have orgasm without intercourse in order to satisfy her without causing pregnancy or destroying her virginity?

PEG: Yes, it is possible. Women can reach orgasm with clitoral, breast, or vaginal stimulation because the clitoris and the folds of skin around the vagina are the most sensitive areas in most women. Again, it is only the first part of the vagina that has a rich supply of nerve endings. Therefore, the male partner can stimulate a woman with his mouth and tongue or his hand. Dry stimulation can be irritating, so saliva or a non-alcohol-containing lotion may be employed as a lubricant to supplement hand stimulation. Again, the woman should feel free to communicate what stimulation excites her most from moment to moment.

MARSHALL: One word of caution: If the man ejaculates at the vaginal opening, it is possible for the sperm to swim into the vagina and into the uterus. That is how virgins become pregnant.

PEG: At the university health clinic, I used to see about one young woman a year who was a virgin with an intact hymen yet who was pregnant. It is not common, but it does occur.

To protect herself against this possibility if she decides she wants to pet to orgasm, a woman might wear a high quality pair of sheer panties and keep them on. They will be nearly as stimulating to the man as her skin would be, and she will have an additional protective barrier to help keep the sperm out of her vagina. But even they are not absolute protection against pregnancy. I did see one virgin who was pregnant who said she had been wearing underpants at the time.

Again, sexual feelings are strong and, therefore, both persons need to be on guard so as not to allow themselves to get into situations that would be too tempting. One couple who had been going together for a couple of years had discussed premarital sex and decided it was not for them. The young man, who was going to another university some miles away, drove to see his girlfriend each weekend, but never stayed overnight. One night there was a big snowstorm, and the roads were totally unsafe when he started to return. He stayed with her, and they had intercourse. The next day they were both in my office, just sick about it; not guilty, but feeling that they had let themselves and each other down, that they had not lived up to what they believed in.

MARSHALL: They failed to do their thing.

Chapter 9
Masturbation

MARSHALL: Masturbation in both the male and female is "fingering" oneself (in the way I defined that before) to the point of sexual excitement or to orgasm. This may be done with the hands or with another object. Men may use some form of sex toy, for example. Women may stimulate the clitoris without involving the vagina, or they may use an object approximately the size and shape of a penis.

Physical Effects of Masturbation

Is masturbation dangerous in terms of physical health, emotional health, or social health? When is it excessive?

MARSHALL: Masturbation has nothing at all to do with physical health. It does not produce insanity, or hair in the palm of the hand, or anything else of that sort. If one engages in masturbation more than the body can take, the body will just fail to respond. Masturbation can only be considered excessive when it or the attendant fantasies interfere with one's reality pursuits, such as working, studying, or dating.

Thoughts While Masturbating

Now, in order to masturbate, most males and females have to have some mental imagery that involves another person. This mental imagery may derive from reading, recalling a story previously read, recalling a previous sexual experience, looking at pornography, or creating a daydream, a fantasy. This fantasy invariably involves another person. This other person may be someone they know or a celebrity, but more commonly is a composite of personality traits and physical attributes. Children are quite egocentric, but we seem to have a built-in requirement that forces us to turn to another person (at least psychologically) for sexual activity after puberty. To achieve orgasm, if that other person is not present in reality, there has to be a daydream creating and involving that other person. This is usually not a daydream of the act of intercourse, but more of foreplay, or attraction. Through the "somebody else" in the fantasy, the individual reaches out and becomes less self-centered psychologically.

Some of the daydreams of patients I have seen cover a wide range, everything from exploits of winning football games, or rescuing a pretty girl from the dragon, or the various modern-day hero types; all the way to the very sick daydreams, the kick-them-in-the-stomach variety or the violent rape. The daydream might take a sadistic or masochistic form; that is, of hurting someone physically or psychologically, or of being hurt.

Guilt

The psychological difficulty with masturbation comes not from the act of masturbation, but from the daydream. If somebody habitually masturbates with a sadistic daydream that he or she is guilty about, he or she is likely to attribute his guilt to the act of masturbation rather than the fantasy. The psychological problems caused will depend on how conflicted he or she is about that particular fantasy.

Some churches consider masturbation per se gravely sinful, which can be a potential source of guilt for the adherent. Apart from the general disapproval of sex historically, there seem to be two basic causes for the continuation of this view. One is the guilt believers have confessed about their masturbation or daydreams, to which the church has reacted by condemning the action. Very likely people have tended to confess the act first; some may never have mentioned the thoughts at all, honestly believing that they had confessed the source of their guilt. The other basis of disapproval of masturbation is social, the perception that one's peers would disapprove. Acknowledgement of the commonality of this practice in popular media, especially through humor, has substantially reduced this concern compared to previous generations.

Female Masturbation

It is quite natural and normal to masturbate. Nearly all men and the majority of women have done it. Sex researcher Kinsey has shown that masturbation persists to some extent throughout married life. With girls, there tends to be a decrease in frequency during late adolescence. Some psychoanalytic theorists have held that a girl masturbates less because of her mortification at not having a penis.

PEG: An idea obviously thought up by a man!

MARSHALL: Two observations apply here. First, the number of women who are masturbating actually increases with age, but of those who do masturbate there is a decrease in the frequency at about age twenty. The number who quit is much less than was previously thought. Second, most women need more than just the daydream; they need the mood and the atmosphere to become sexually aroused in order to masturbate successfully.

Interestingly, sometimes when a person is "lovesick," he is not able to use masturbation for a release of sexual tension. The reason is that once the daydream gets started and the sexual feelings really mount, the daydream switches to real memories of the loved person and continues as reminiscences, or future hopes, while the old standard masturbatory daydream is lost from attention.

Most men and women continue to masturbate in married life; usually when their spouse is unavailable because of travel, menstruation, or perhaps an argument. Likewise, some women who have had an active sexual life and have then been divorced or widowed seem to experience a chronic sexual tension which they can release by masturbation.

Nocturnal Emission

What is a nocturnal emission?

Nocturnal emission is a phenomenon that occurs in males after puberty. When there is a build-up of excess semen that is not released by masturbation or intercourse, the body gets rid of it with an ejaculation during sleep, a "wet dream." (See "Nocturnal Emissions" in Chapter 17.)

Chapter 10
Feeling, Thinking, and Doing

MARSHALL: As Peggy said, you are not responsible for your feelings; you are only partially responsible for your thoughts, but you are entirely responsible for your actions.

The law—except for the laws of conspiracy, motivation, and intent—takes only actions into account. You can plan a man's murder, buy the gun, and draw a detailed diagram of your plan, but until you step up and take aim, they cannot arrest you for attempted murder. Religion goes one step further. It places negative sanctions on the active process of thinking as well as on doing. All the world's major religions condemn your harboring hatred, dwelling on wrongs done to you, or wishing to do wrong. "Thou shalt not covet" is added after "Thou shalt not steal." But none of the major religions places a negative sanction on feelings. There is no commandment against being aroused when you see your neighbor's spouse. Action, thought, and feeling are all positively sanctioned; that is, thou shalt love thy… But religion stops short of negative sanctions on feelings, or the thought that accompanies the feeling, unless it is dwelt on.

No one can control his feelings entirely. If we could, no one would ever feel embarrassed. An individual who feels scared or eerie when walking through a graveyard at night cannot stop feeling scared by wishing to, or by thinking, "There are no such things as ghosts; I have no reason to be fearful." Even if he acts happy by whistling, he will still feel scared. But he can control his actions and get out of the graveyard and thereby indirectly control his feelings. It is only the neurotic who places negative sanctions (guilt) on his own spontaneous feelings. You can learn a good deal about yourself by noting what type of situation produces what type of feeling, and how you act in response to the feeling.

Usually feeling, thinking, and acting are fairly synchronous, forming a harmonious whole. Many of the sexual problems people have are due to a lack of this harmony. Feelings are out of harmony in such varied conditions and situations as impotence, frigidity, rape, and sexual deviation. Thinking is out of harmony when an individual violates his or her own value system or does not take steps to prevent contraception when pregnancy is not desired. Acting is rarely out of phase if feeling and thinking are in harmony. If the other two are at odds, as is often the case, the action will probably be a compromise.

Sexual Feelings Only

The act of sex can be carried out with a multitude of different feelings and combinations of feelings.

Prostitute-relationship

MARSHALL: Prostitutes and gigolos and the customers who patronize them have little or no feelings for their partners as individuals. The male customer is almost exclusively interested in ejaculation, and money is the primary interest of most of the sellers. For the man, it is hedonistic—more pleasurable—to use someone else's body rather than his own hands to masturbate with. The dynamics of his relationship tend to consist of feelings of superiority and of dominating his sexual partner. He chooses a partner, uses him or her, and then can cast him or her aside with utter disregard. The seller most often feels superior to the men as suckers and fools. Hence, if for the prostitute there is a premium on speed of performance, then the individual personality of the customer must necessarily count for little. The partners are readily substituted for each other; any paying customer will do. This is the same type of relationship most animals have with their copulatory partners, although many also take mates and relate to their mates as individuals. Women who hire gigolos tend to seek atmosphere that culminates in sex: an escort, a romantic dinner, maybe some dancing, an opportunity to feel desired and desirable, no matter how artificial; but ultimately the seller's role avoids personal feelings in lieu of moving on after satisfying his customer.

The Other Extreme

At the other extreme is the man who cares so much about his partner's feelings that whenever he perceives (correctly or not) that she really does not want intercourse even though she is cooperating, he either has a premature ejaculation or is unable to maintain an erection sufficient to insert his penis. This problem is not uncommon.

Rapists

Men who commit forceful rape often are "acting out" an unusual combination of feelings. Intercourse with consenting women may be available at the time of the rape to the majority of these men. Instead, they commit the act of rape with a need to engender feelings of fear and helplessness in a woman and feelings of power and superiority in themselves in combination with their sexual feelings.

Nymphomaniacs

Are some women nymphs?

Yes, they are another example of action springing from an unusual combination of feelings, but they are very, very few. It seems a man is apt to call a particular woman a nymph just because she has a greater sex drive than he has. There are also many women who do not quite achieve orgasm with intercourse and are left with a high degree of pelvic congestion and sexual tension. Often they seek to relieve their feelings by repeated intercourse. This situation may develop into a chronic cycle. The true nymphomaniac has a compulsion to engage in intercourse. As in other compulsions, the compulsive act itself is only a symbol, an unconscious symbol of one (or several) ambivalent and conflictive unconscious feelings. In nymphomania, the unconscious feeling or meaning attached to the act of intercourse is not sex, but something neurotically more important to the woman.

Is this always psychological?

MARSHALL: There is that absolute word "always." For all practical purposes, it is always psychological. I know of two cases of nymphomania reported in medical literature which were associated with and supposedly due to a tumor in a particular area of the brain.

Perversions

What constitutes moral actions as opposed to perversions in the sex act?

MARSHALL: Perversion means a turning from the natural to the unnatural. Psychiatrically defined, a perverse sex act is an act between two people where the habitually preferred method of stimulation for greater enjoyment is obtained from some form of stimulation other than that provided by the penis in the vagina. If other activities are used for variety or for foreplay to the usual sex act, they are not considered perversions.

PEG: I think that for an act to be considered moral it has to be mutually agreeable to the couple and not hurtful or deceitful to others.

MARSHALL: Yes, that is part of what I think morality is in sex: acts that are acceptable and enjoyable to both people and that are not performed by one without consideration of the other partner's enjoyment. Psychiatry does not have a category of "perversions." They are called sexual deviations; that is, deviations (or departures) from the norm or average. This is a much better term in that it is free of moral or legal connotations. The deviant group includes nymphomaniacs, transvestites, exhibitionists, pedophiles, sadists, masochists, and others. Difficulties arise when religious or moral principles are written into the law. Consideration shifts from acts to people, and the people become perverts rather than just the act being perverted. The habitual aspect is completely lost.

Two people can also satisfy each other in a deviant way, but I do not think society has a right to complain about it. It can be unnatural, but I do not think it should be illegal. These distinctions should be kept clear; that is, it is not necessarily a good practice to mix morality with legality. If two adults are involved in deviant behavior that harms nobody else and confine their activities to private places, there is no victim. Why then should it be a crime? Where the only legal concern is the enforcement of a morality, the application of the law *always* results in socio-economic injustice.

Like nymphomania, many perversions begin as a symbolic act with a degree of compulsion, usually to reduce anxiety. The act is found enjoyable initially or after some experience and, since it combines both sex and relief of anxiety, it becomes preferred. In time, the symbolic aspect may become negligible. If abstinence from the act produces anxiety, and if the patient will abstain, psychiatry can most often produce a change.

Homosexuality

Is that true for homosexuals?

MARSHALL: Possibly. If an individual seeks homosexual outlets when he is under pressure or tension, or when experiencing fear or something he cannot define, and furthermore, if he will abstain from homosexual activity, then psychiatry sometimes can revert him to heterosexual functioning. On the other hand, if homosexuals seek help under the pressure of a court, a boss, or their spouses without internal motivation, then psychiatry can do little in the way of increasing their heterosexual interests. Many psychiatrists will work with the latter type of homosexuals to help them deal with the reality of pressures from the outside. Of course, there are many homosexuals who are satisfied with their way of life and neither want nor need help.

What do homosexuals do?

In men, the most common form of homosexual activity is one man stimulating the other by mouth-genital contact. This is called *fellatio*. It is usually carried to the point of orgasm. Stimulation may be simultaneous. The sexual stimulation may also be obtained by the penis in the rectum of the partner; this is called *anal sex* or *sodomy*. These terms are also applied to stimulation obtained by the penis in a woman's rectum.

In women, the most common form of sexual activity is mouth stimulation of the clitoris. This is called *cunnilingus*. It also may be done simultaneously. The term also applies to a man using his mouth to stimulate a woman's genitals. Sometimes one woman may stimulate her partner with an artificial penis called a *dildo*. The dildo may be strapped on her pelvis or held in her hand. The psychological relationship and hence the sexual behavior that precedes the genital stimulation is as varied as it is in heterosexual relationships.

What causes a person to be a homosexual?

MARSHALL: I do not think anyone really knows. Homosexuality appears to be a generic term applied to several entities rather than a single one. There are three recognized patterns of relationships between a child and his (or her) parents that seem causative.

(These are described in Chapter 18.) There is also some evidence that if a boy or girl in the early teens has an enjoyable and satisfying homosexual relationship with an older person, then he or she is apt to develop a homosexual orientation. This is not true if the homosexual relationship is with a peer.

There is also the unfortunate teenager who is discovered in a homosexual act with a peer. Research has documented that most heterosexuals have had at least one homosexual or quasi-homosexual experience during adolescence. Being caught in a fleeting moment of experimentation can lead to being branded by the adults as a homosexual. This stamping of an identity before the adolescent has had a chance to explore several identities is a serious injustice that may do irrevocable harm. Adolescents who appear somewhat effeminate or tomboyish due to delayed puberty or who have a certain physique may also be wrongly labeled as homosexuals. Others have such a complete homosexual orientation that they perceive themselves as the opposite sex. They are called *transsexuals*. If they undergo surgical reassignment, they are called *transgender*.

A large number of female homosexuals (*lesbians*) do not have any homosexual thoughts or feelings until their thirties or forties. Most of these women have normal psychiatric histories, and do not seem to have had significant marital problems either of a sexual or non-sexual nature.

How should you respond when a homosexual approaches you?

That depends on your own inclinations. But assuming you are not favorably predisposed, what about a simple "No, thanks"? Someone who is not your "type" finding you attractive does not reflect on you. That is to say, receiving invitations does not indicate you are homosexual, but it does suggest you might be sending sexual messages. Someone getting mixed or misleading signals from you should lead you to reflect on why that happens, and whether or not you want to change your behavior.

What is a latent homosexual?

MARSHALL: Since the term "latent homosexual" is applied so indiscriminately, it usually means nothing except that the individual is not an active homosexual. Strictly applied, it refers to an individual who has an aversion to the opposite sex or whose sexual fantasies involve homosexual relationships. Some latent homosexuals have fairly normal heterosexual fantasies that shift to homosexual content as they near orgasm. Latent homosexuality may also be evidenced by feelings of panic or anxiety at the very thought of being a homosexual. Most often the thought is triggered by a homosexual proposition and may result in an attack on the solicitor or an acute panicky need to have heterosexual intercourse for self-reassurance.

Oral-genital Contact

Do married people try oral intercourse? Are you frigid if you will not try?

PEG: If oral-genital contact is unacceptable and unaesthetic to you, there is no reason to do it. Some couples and some individuals find it enjoyable, and some couples do not. Frigidity does not enter into it; it is a personal preference. Do not ever feel you have to prove anything in a love relationship. For many couples, not only is it an enjoyable and stimulating method of arousing the partner, it is also enjoyed in its own right. After all, mouth stimulation is enjoyed in many other forms, such as kissing, smoking, chewing gum, etc. As for the cleanliness aspect, assuming the couples bathe regularly, the mouth is far more contaminated by various bacteria than are the genitals. Also oral-genital contact is one way to be physically intimate and achieve orgasm without any risk of pregnancy.

How common is oral-genital contact in married life?

MARSHALL: Kinsey first reported in the 1940s that 60 percent of college graduate couples have had one experience with it. Of this 60 percent, the wife reciprocates in about 47 percent of the cases. Interestingly, the level of education is a variant here. The incidence with high school graduates falls to 20 percent and with high school dropouts it is 11 percent. Subsequent research shows those numbers rising somewhat. Research also shows the practice becoming more common among unmarried adolescents, which suggests it may become more prevalent among married couples in the future.

What is sixty-nine?

MARSHALL: Sixty-nine refers to simultaneous stimulation of both partners' genitals with each other's mouths. The term is derived from the similarity of the position of the bodies of the partners to each other compared with the position of the two numerals in 69. The main connotation is homosexual activity, but it may also be simultaneous heterosexual oral-genital stimulation—the genital kiss.

Chapter 11
Menstruation

The Menstrual Cycle

PEG: Menstruation is the process of a woman's body eliminating unneeded reproductive material. The lining of the uterus builds up a thick, succulent layer of blood and nutrients for a fertilized egg. If no egg is fertilized, no hormones are released, and as the hormone levels fall, the lining is shed over a period of several days through the cervix and vagina as the menstrual flow. Then the process of preparation for a fertilized egg begins again. This cycle repeats itself once every twenty-one to thirty-five days, with most women having a twenty-eight to thirty-day cycle. A few women have a very regular cycle; others vary by two to six days. Illness, emotional tension, and any number of other things can modify the length of the cycle. (For a discussion of ovulation in the menstrual cycle, see "The Rhythm Method" in Chapter 12.)

Arousal at the Time of Ovulation

Is a girl more easily aroused at the time of ovulation?

PEG: It has been said that there is some increased sexual desire at the time of ovulation. There is definitely a hormonal shift, and this could well account for the supposed change. On the other hand, there seems to be a great deal of variability and individuality among women.

MARSHALL: Several studies have been published on this question. Those based solely on a single interview are anything but conclusive. In several longer-term studies, it was discovered that women, in general, pay little attention to their level of desire, at least consciously, and many had to be instructed about how to recognize sexual feelings. Actually, when it was pointed out that sexual feelings could be recognized by "dreams of a sexual nature, a desire to be close to someone, a desire to be held, genital sensations, a feeling of being feminine, a yearning for love, a feeling of helplessness, and others, they expressed surprise." The report added: "Some women even believed such sensations were sinful or 'not nice'." In short, of the three or four prospective studies on the subject, all have found a significant increase in sexual desire on the thirteenth day and just at the end of menstruation. Presumably intercourse on the thirteenth day would result in the sperm being near the egg at the time of ovulation (fourteenth day). We also know that for pregnancy to occur the egg must be fertilized in the upper third of the oviduct. In any event, play it safe by being prepared.

Premenstrual Tension

What is PMS?

PEG: Some women get psychologically upset just before their periods. They become very emotional; we call it emotional liability. If you just look at them cross-eyed, they might burst into tears, or explode in an angry tirade. Recently this has been attributed to the hormonal shifts that go on during the menstrual cycle. For three, four, or five days prior to the start of the menstrual flow, some women have a marked retention of water within the body. As soon as the hormone level falls and they menstruate, the excess water is excreted via the kidneys as urine; but, before that happens, some of these women will gain three to six pounds of excess weight. They may increase an inch or two around the waist and they may get ankle swelling. The water is within the cells themselves, not between cells or in the bloodstream. It has been proven that just as the water gets into the cells of the waist and ankles, it also gets into the brain cells. The brain cells actually become edematous and swollen, causing the headaches, tension, and the emotional liability we call premenstrual tension or premenstrual syndrome—PMS. We can treat this condition, and many over-the-counter remedies are available without prescription. Many women take medicine for four to five days each month, beginning when they start feeling the premenstrual tension, and this handles the symptoms very nicely. We might describe the cause of premenstrual tension then as a hormonally-produced retention of fluids within the cells of the body, most importantly in the brain.

Intercourse During Menstruation

Can you have intercourse on your "flow" days?

PEG: Yes, you can have intercourse during menstruation. It is kind of messy and just not very aesthetic for some couples, but there is no health hazard in it.

Onset of Menstruation

How old should a girl be before she starts worrying about not yet having her first period?

The onset of menarche varies widely. For most girls, this is between the ages of ten and fifteen, but many do start sooner or later. A girl is never too young or old to express concerns to her physician, who is best able to determine the status of her health and development.

Chapter 12
Contraception

A Basis for Comparison

PEG: Many questions we receive are on the subject of contraception: What contraceptive methods are available and what are their various efficacy rates? I think this should be basic knowledge. The basis I will use for comparing the efficacy rates of contraceptives is a formula that 85 out of 100 women in the fertile age range having an active sex life and using no contraceptives at all will become pregnant in a year's time. Whether the pregnancy is carried to term is not a function of the contraceptive used; it depends on many other factors.

The Douche

The least effective method of contraception is *the douche*. This is just washing out the vagina after intercourse. Douching does not significantly reduce pregnancy rates. In fact, immediate use after vaginal sex may push sperm deeper into the uterus, thus encouraging a pregnancy. However, it also increases the risk of inflammatory disease as well as a potentially very dangerous ectopic pregnancy. It makes no difference whether water, vinegar, or a commercial douching product is used. The female reproductive system naturally cleanses itself, so douching for personal hygiene is not necessary.

The Rhythm Method

Another common method of contraception is the *rhythm method*. This is abstinence from intercourse during the time when a woman thinks that she is ovulating. This method has a pregnancy rate of about 12 to 22 women per 100 per year, and is the only birth control practice currently approved by the Roman Catholic Church. Using the rhythm method, the "unsafe" period is about three to four days before the date of ovulation through three to four days after that date. The ovulation date can most easily be determined retrospectively. A woman ovulates fourteen days before her menstruation starts. She always knows in retrospect when she ovulates, but it is hard for her to gauge ahead of time unless her periods are very regular. If a woman has a period very regularly every twenty-eight days, she should ovulate on approximately the fourteenth day; if she has a thirty-day cycle, she ovulates on the sixteenth day, and so on.

MARSHALL: If she has an irregular cycle, she ovulates on an irregular day.

PEG: For women who have irregular periods or whose periods are readily upset by emotional upheaval, minor illness, or any type of stress, the rhythm method is a particularly difficult type of contraception to use efficaciously. Statistically the odds may be helped by averaging the length of the last three cycles. A basal temperature chart also increases the efficacy of the rhythm method.

Basal Temperature

Would you explain basal temperature, please?

A woman's *basal temperature*, her temperature on first awakening (before she gets out of bed, or starts worrying, or before anything else) rises about one degree at the time of ovulation. About a day before ovulating, there is a slight dip in basal temperature. However, the dip can be missed, and then the rise appears to be less than a degree.

If you usually menstruate regularly but have been under stress for two weeks, when would you ovulate?

PEG: Fourteen days before you menstruate. That is the difficulty in using this method. Furthermore, sperm can fertilize an egg as much as 48 hours after intercourse. They have been found alive in the vagina 72 hours after intercourse; hence, some doctors say 72 hours instead of 48. How long you abstain before or after your calculated ovulation date will depend on your conservatism. Some couples wait two days on either side, some three or four. This will vary with your conservatism, and your efficacy will vary with that, too.

Coitus Interruptus

Another method in common use is *coitus interruptus*. With this method the man withdraws his penis prior to the time he ejaculates. Coitus interruptus has a pregnancy rate overall of about 15 to 16 women per 100 per year when this is used as the sole method of contraception. Especially in teens and young adults, this is a poor, poor method of contraception. To be used successfully, coitus interruptus requires that the male partner have self-knowledge; that he know himself well enough to sense the beginning of his orgasmic experience to be able to withdraw in time. The other problem with this method is that, prior to the major ejaculation in the man, there is some involuntary emission of fluid (semen) which is uncontrollable and which he is unaware of. This semen contains live sperm. So, even if he withdraws prior to the major ejaculation, it is possible that he can leave some live sperm in the vagina.

The Diaphragm

A device for contraception with the rate of about 6 to 16 pregnancies per 100 per year is the diaphragm. It is a pliable ring with a dome-shaped piece of plastic or rubber stretched across it. It is inserted into the vagina, much like a tampon, and fits over the cervix, the opening of the uterus into the vagina. Supposedly it blocks the passage of sperm from the vagina through the cervix into the uterus. A physician must fit the diaphragm to ensure that it is the proper size. The wide range of efficacy is most probably due to improper insertion by the user, either due to lack of instruction or carelessness.

Intravaginal Preparations

The intravaginal preparations—the jellies, creams, or foams—have a pregnancy rate of about 8 to 29 women per 100 per year. The preparations have to be used with each act of intercourse and, like the diaphragm, they should not be disturbed for about eight hours after intercourse. Intravaginal cream and a diaphragm are usually used together, rimming the diaphragm with the cream and also putting some in the center of the diaphragm. This brings the diaphragm's efficacy to the rate of the vaginal cream or jelly alone. However, using the diaphragm with the cream does not reduce the pregnancy rate any further. It appears to be just as efficacious to use either the foam, or the jelly, or the cream by itself. The jellies, creams, and foams, which can be purchased at regular drugstores without a prescription, work by immobilizing or killing the sperm. The foam is believed to give somewhat greater protection than either the jelly or the cream or the combination of diaphragm and jelly.

The Condom

Another contraceptive is the condom, also called a prophylactic, a safety, or a rubber. This is a narrow balloon-like rubber sack that is put over the erect penis and worn during intercourse. It catches the semen which contains the sperm, thus preventing them from being deposited in the vagina. The condom has a pregnancy rate of between 8 to 15 women per 100 per year, depending on which report you read. The pregnancies are due primarily either to the condom breaking in some way or slipping off within the vagina and spilling the collected semen. A condom may break because of an air bubble which is caused usually by a partial loss of the erection before or during intercourse. The penis must be withdrawn fairly promptly following ejaculation or its shrinkage may allow the condom to slip off, or leak intravaginally. It might be worth mentioning that, whatever its faults, the condom is the only contraceptive device which also prevents the transmission of venereal disease. Condoms can be purchased in a drugstore without prescription and are manufactured with and without added lubricant or a spermicide.

Combo

You will note the condom and the foam utilize entirely different means of interfering with the process of conception. Each has a pregnancy rate as low as 8 percent. If both methods are utilized simultaneously, the pregnancy rate is as low as 1 percent.

The Intrauterine Contraceptive Device

(Coil or Loop)

Next, we want to mention the intrauterine contraceptive device— the coil or loop—which has a pregnancy rate of about 3 women per 100 per year. The device, which must be inserted in the uterus by a physician, is not usually satisfactory in women who have not already had a baby. Frequently cramps and excessive bleeding from the uterus may occur with this device. Some women are so uncomfortable with these devices that their bodies expel them or they must have them removed. Theoretically, this device causes an increased motility in the fallopian tubes so that, even if an egg is fertilized, it moves along at a faster than normal rate and reaches the uterine cavity too immature to implant itself. We do not know why the device sometimes fails.

The Pill

The contraceptive pill, which is available only by prescription in the USA, is of two basic kinds, the combination and the sequential. The sequential pill has a pregnancy rate of 2 to 3 women per 100 per year; the combination type pill has a pregnancy rate of virtually zero.

The pills are composed of two normal female hormones, called estrogen and progestin. The combination pills have both estrogen and progestin in each day's dose. In the sequential pill only the estrogen is taken for about the first sixteen days; then a combination of the estrogen and progestin is taken for the last five to six days, depending on the brand.

The pills work in at least three different ways. First, they set up a hormonal balance similar to a normal pregnancy. Pregnant women do not get one pregnancy on top of another. Since the pills cause the ovaries to react as though you were pregnant, the ovaries do not release any ovum ("egg"); that is, the pills prevent ovulation. Second, they cause the cervix (the opening of the uterus into the vagina) to produce a thick tenacious mucus which the sperm are unable to penetrate. Thus, the ova in the uterus or above it are protected from fertilization. Third, the pills keep the lining of the uterus from becoming very thick; therefore, it is not nutrient enough to sustain a fertilized egg should one embed itself. The relative thinness of the uterine lining causes the menstrual flow to be less than usual while a woman is on the pill. Thus, there are three known ways in which the pill prevents conception, and that is probably why this method is so successful.

What happens if you forget a pill?

PEG: In general, the early days of the cycle are the most important. If it is the fifth or sixth day, the chances of pregnancy go up considerably. If you remember within the next day, take the pill as soon as you can. If you forget for twenty-four hours, take two pills together. If you forget for more than twenty-four hours, you can take two pills when you remember, but you had better use an additional method of contraception the remainder of that month.

Can women regulate when they are going to menstruate?

PEG: When women have a period while they are on the pill, it is because they have stopped taking the pill. The pill is used cyclically: a woman starts taking the pill on the fifth day of her menstrual cycle, counting day number one the fifth day there is any menstrual flow. She takes the pill every day for twenty or twenty-one days and then stops. Usually two to three days after she has stopped, she will begin her period. That is day number one of the next cycle, and on day number five she starts on her pills again. Actually, if the woman finds out she always has her period two days after she has taken the pill, and this is going to be a special weekend or some other special occasion, then she can take pills a few days longer without interruption. In effect, women can regulate their periods and have them when they want them when using the pill. This is a fringe benefit, and is much easier with the combination pill rather than the sequential.

Are there side effects from using the pill?

PEG: There are many possible side effects with the pill. Some women starting out on the pills go through some of the early signs of pregnancy, such as morning nausea and vomiting, and fluid retention and breast tenderness. Another side effect that occurs with the pill is weight gain, which can be of two types. One is fluid retention similar to what some women get just before they menstruate. Their ankles, hands, and abdomens swell. The other is a real increase in body mass. It is difficult to determine for sure just what is the cause of the weight gain in some women. In certain instances, there are apparently real weight gains perhaps due to increased efficiency in absorption of food by the intestines. Other possible side effects of the pill are depression and headaches. Some have reported a decreased sexual desire. The FDA requires that potential side effects be spelled out clearly in writing. You should discuss any concerns with your prescribing physician. Also you should *never* take birth-control or any other kind of medication prescribed for someone else.

The "Morning-after Pill"

What is the pill we can take to prevent pregnancy after having sex?

The treatment commonly called the "morning-after pill" is RU-486, also known generically as mifepristone. An artificial steroid, it blocks progesterone, a hormone needed to continue pregnancy. A second drug, a prostaglandin (usually misoprostol in the USA) is given approximately 48 hours later to increase its effectiveness.

RU-486 does not prevent pregnancy, but rather terminates pregnancy after contraception. Technically, it is an abortion (See Chapter 14), but is usually thought of as birth control, perhaps because it does not involve surgical abortion, and because it is used at the embryonic stage prior to obvious evidence of pregnancy. The two-drug treatment is necessary because the first causes complete abortion only about 60% of the time. The second drug causes uterine contractions to help expel the embryo, thus increasing the effectiveness to approximately 92% through the seventh week of pregnancy. In most cases the process takes between two days and two weeks, but it can take up to three or even four weeks.

Like all drug treatments, use of RU-486 may cause symptoms and does carry risks. Common symptoms include nausea, severe cramps, dizziness, vomiting, diarrhea, and heavy bleeding. Several cases of death due to untreated sepsis have been reported.

Physician supervision is recommended when using RU-486, even if the laws and requirements of your jurisdiction are less restrictive. Patients should have access to emergency facilities and the presence of a helpful friend or family member during the first few days when excessive bleeding is possible.

While it is called "morning-after," RU-486 is considered safest and most effective up to—but not exceeding—the 49th day after conception. Regardless of when it is used, a pelvic exam is strongly recommended, as there are several conditions such as ectopic pregnancy where RU-486 should not be used.

Waiting until after contraception to deal with pregnancy issues carries both moral and medical implications. Effective use of other forms of birth control that prevent contraception is always preferred.

The Sterilization Operation

MARSHALL: A sterilization operation is a safe and efficient method for both the male and the female. However, the operation is not always reversible, so a person needs to contemplate his or her feelings should circumstances change the desire to have children.

PEG: Technically the operation is much simpler in the male than in the female. The vasa deferentia, the two tubes that carry sperm from the testes, are cut. This is called *vasectomy*. The operation is done under local anesthesia and can be done in a doctor's office. In the female the fallopian tubes are cut. This is called *tubal ligation* or "tubes tied." This requires an abdominal operation under general anesthesia. Hence, it must be done in a hospital.

After a man is sterilized, does he have an ejaculation?

MARSHALL: Oh yes, the ejaculation will still contain secretions from the prostate gland and seminal vesicles. Because some sperm are stored in the reproductive tract, it takes about ten ejaculations after the operation before the semen is devoid of sperm. But the operation in no way interferes with potency, sex drive, hormones, or other sexual characteristics. You can have intercourse the night of the operation.

A Summary of Contraception

The effectiveness rates we have been describing are intended to give you approximate comparisons of different methods. Rates will vary at different times in different populations participating in different studies. Effectiveness rates also depend substantially on how consistently and properly birth-control methods are used. Rarely is any method requiring ongoing use practiced correctly all the time.

Without emphasizing the actual numbers, consider this summary of common methods ranked, as we see them, as most effective to least effective:

Abstinence is always effective. Permanent sterilization such as tubal ligation and vasectomy are nearly always effective, though some failures have been reported. IUDs and injections such as Depo Provera are highly effective. Drug therapies such as "the pill," "the patch," and NuvaRing are highly effective. Continuous breastfeeding tends to reduce pregnancy rates to about five out of 100 women per year. Natural family planning methods vary widely, but if practiced faithfully, can be next-most effective. Barrier methods such as sponges, cervical caps, spermicides, diaphragms, female condoms, and male condoms are effective, but their rates vary widely depending on how carefully and consistently they are used. Douching may actually increase chances of pregnancy slightly, as well as risk of complications.

Many birth-control methods offer the additional benefit of protection from *sexually transmitted diseases (STDs)*. Both pregnancy prevention and STD protection are especially important when sexual partners are not involved in an ongoing, monogamous, committed, caring relationship.

The consequences of poor birth-control planning are potentially life-changing. An important part of being sufficiently mature to have sexual relations with a partner of the opposite sex is being sufficiently mature to take responsibility for both contraception and the consequences should there be a pregnancy. Adolescents eager for sexual experiences are especially vulnerable to unplanned pregnancies at a time in their lives when they are likely least prepared to assume the responsibilities.

Chapter 13
Pregnancy and Alternatives to Parenthood

Signs of Pregnancy

How can you tell if you are pregnant, and when should a pregnant woman begin seeing a doctor?

PEG: Usually the first clue is a missed menstrual period. As a rule, the period should be eight to ten days overdue before pregnancy is seriously suspected. When the second period is also missed, the probability of pregnancy increases a great deal. However, it is not uncommon for a woman to have one or two episodes of bloody discharge simulating menstruation during the first third of a pregnancy. The breasts frequently become larger and tender. Nausea and vomiting, especially in the morning, are also common signs. One further sign is a desire for frequent urination. Over-the-counter pregnancy tests available at any drugstore are quite reliable indicators, though not 100 percent.

Seeing the Doctor

In regard to the second part of your question, a woman should be seen as early in the pregnancy as possible, and then at four-week intervals until the seventh month; the next two months she should be seen every two weeks, and weekly during the ninth month. Prenatal care is important to ensure optimal health of both the mother and the baby.

MARSHALL: Many do not see a doctor as soon as you should. However, if you notice your ankles swelling up in the evenings (they may not be swollen in the mornings), see a doctor right away. The only other symptom you might notice is a burning sensation on urination, which is a sign of bladder infection. That needs prompt attention anytime.

Options with Pregnancy

PEG: Too many young, unmarried women find themselves unintentionally pregnant, so they see this as a reason to hurry and get married. I usually counsel against this unless the two are deeply committed to each other, or are engaged and had marital plans prior to their suspecting that she is pregnant. Certainly, being pregnant out of wedlock is not easy, but it only lasts nine months. Marriage to someone you do not love lasts a lot longer. Frequently, such couples try to make it work and have one or two other children before they break up the marriage.

MARSHALL: Divorce is particularly rough on the children of couples who married because of pregnancy. Along with the minor problems that come up in the marriage, they frequently wonder if, had she not been pregnant, would they have married or not. This is an area fraught with hazard. It is hard on the child, too, both directly and indirectly. The parents may resent the child, perhaps indirectly communicating, "You're really the cause of it all; if you hadn't existed then we would have found someone better and been happier." Often, marriage is not a happy solution.

Adoption

PEG: Another alternative is to carry the baby to term and give it up for adoption. For some, this is a particularly good way of handling the situation. They know they have made some couple immeasurably happy by this child and can feel that this was the best solution to the problem.

However, there are some who elect this route and do not come out feeling like this at all. Some of them find out whether they had a boy or girl, and some do not decide on adoption immediately but keep the baby the two to five days they are in the hospital before they give up the child. I talked with a woman who delivered four years ago and knows she had a blond boy. Every time she sees a blond four-year-old boy on the street, she immediately starts to wonder if that is her child. Young women like this suffer immeasurably. They keep hounding themselves incessantly. For them it is clearly not an easy way out. If you are going to allow the baby to be adopted, it is important to try to decide before delivery so that it will be easier on you. The adoption agency will then have enough time to locate a suitable home and have it ready by the time of delivery. If you have any ambivalence about the decision, before or after, please talk to a counselor who specializes in this area.

Keeping the Baby

Another alternative that some elect is to carry the baby to term, then keep it but not get married. The mother assumes a tremendous responsibility in this situation, often requiring assistance with childcare and/or financial support. She also needs to ensure the child has regular contact with the father or a suitable male role model. In most cases, having a child out of wedlock will substantially limit options and opportunities, from education to career to relationships.

Placement of the Baby

A risky situation a mother can place her child in is to give it to her own parents to raise. The child grows up confused as to who his mother is. Does he have two mothers, or is his sister sometimes his sister and sometimes his mother; and which mother has the "final say"? For example, a mother at delivery may give her baby to her parents temporarily—that is, until she can make a home for the child. As the months go by, further arrangements are usually put off until after she enters a committed relationship such as marriage. If such temporary arrangements are to be made, they should not last longer than five or six months. Under no circumstances should the child be separated from his functioning mother between the ages of six months and fourteen months. No time is a good time to lose a functioning mother. But any time during six to fourteen months and ages three to seven is probably worse than any time during fourteen months to three years or after age seven.

Even permanent placements of this type seldom work out since there is a natural tendency for the mother to want the child back at a later date, especially if she moves away.

If grandparents are to keep the child, they should always be known as grandparents, never as parents. The problem then frequently arises as to "Who is mother and father, and why aren't they looking after me?" This hurts, especially when mother is around once or twice a week but is uninvolved. Still, it is better than the effects on the child that occur where there is role confusion.

Chapter 14
Abortion

Abortion

Abortion is the surgical termination of pregnancy, resulting in removal and death of the fetus, usually long before the fetus would have matured sufficiently to survive apart from its mother. The legality of abortion varies widely around the world, country to country, and from region to region within countries. It ranges from strictly prohibited and harshly punished to being available on demand, albeit with limitations and restriction. In some areas, the procedure is legal only under certain government-specified conditions. Abortion raises many issues, including morality, religion, civil rights, psychology, and health.

Do many girls have to have a hysterectomy because of an abortion?

PEG: No. A hysterectomy is surgical removal of the uterus. Abortion could lead to a hysterectomy if the bleeding cannot be stopped or if subsequent infection could not be controlled. Occasionally, instead of just scraping out the lining of the uterus, which is the procedure for most abortions, the physician's instrument breaches the wall of the uterus. However, it would be rare that a hysterectomy would have to be done because of this. The primary problem is infection, and this is usually handled by repeating the scraping, trying to get at all the infected areas, and administering high doses of antibiotics. The main point is that anyone who has had an abortion should seek medical help promptly at the first suspicion that something might not be just right.

Reasons for an Abortion

Most women who undergo abortion want at least one child at a later time. Some want never to have children. A young woman may not want to deliver her first pregnancy for one of several reasons: insufficient financial means, her young age, desire for education, expectations of future marriage, neurosis, being on the verge of divorce, or strong desire not to share parenthood with the father. If she is forced to have this unwanted child, she may never experience the joy of a wanted child. The unwanted child is more likely to have problems. Children acutely sense when they are unwanted, especially if they are unloved. Parenting presents many challenges among the moments of wonder and joy, so a mother who is unwilling or unable to rise to such a level of responsibility should not subject an innocent child to harms ranging from indifference to hostility. A woman who chooses abortion recognizes that she is not ready to be a mother, and that she is unable or unwilling to commit to full-term pregnancy and adoption.

Illegal Abortion

Many areas of the world either make abortion illegal, or erect so many barriers that illegal abortion becomes an attractive option. Illegal abortion can be traumatic psychologically and physically. A woman who goes to an illegal abortionist is not in a position to question his or her credentials, training, experience, or access to facilities. Usually she is not sure whether or not the instruments are indeed surgical, much less sterile. Very serious complications can result from illegal abortions, including death. In addition to infection, there is the risk during illegal abortion of perforating the uterus. The further along the pregnancy, the greater the risk. Many criminal abortionists will not operate on a woman who is more than eight weeks pregnant (usually ten weeks since last menstrual period). Twelve weeks of pregnancy is the limit for most; the danger of perforation increases significantly at that time.

Abortions performed in a hospital are often performed up to twenty weeks of pregnancy.

Psychological Effects of Illegal Abortion

Aside from the physical danger, there is a traumatic psychological aspect to illegal abortion. For example, a woman may be blindfolded and taken to a secret location. The inappropriate setting and unsanitary conditions can render her scared of mistakes and complications. Fear of detection and social or legal reprisals can lead to stress for an extended period. If the abortionist did not carry the authoritative air of a qualified physician, the patient may be left feeling physically violated. For many, the mere fact of committing an illegal act leaves them feeling they have done something wrong, possibly adding doubts after already having made a difficult decision.

MARSHALL: It is not just the women who may have psychiatric complications because of an abortion, but men can, too. Take this case history of a military man who came to me when he was twenty-eight years old. He had been fairly active sexually in the United States before going overseas, where he was also active sexually. When he found out later that his overseas partner got an abortion, he was convinced the child was his. He said, "She had no right to kill my son." This man, who was not a Catholic and was not religious in any of the usual senses of the word, was really shaken by the experience. He had not been aware anything like this would disturb him at all. From then until I saw him seven years later, he was impotent. He could masturbate, and he could maintain an erection, but when he would introduce his penis into the vagina of a woman, he would lose his erection. He finally decided to seek medical help when he found a woman he genuinely loved and wanted to marry. I worked with him for a short time. He got married and has not had difficulty.

Thus, you really have to know yourself and examine your whole system. You should consider what the various consequences of your actions would really mean to you. "To your own self be true."

The Abortion Debate

The arguments for and against abortion-on-request boil down to the rights of the state, the rights of the fetus, and the rights of the pregnant woman—with the moral issues and religious sanctions attached to all three. The moral and religious sanctions of the rights of the state are the least well recognized.

Role of Religion in Society

Organized religion has many functions in a society; a major one is generating a feeling of group solidarity. As such, respect for and preservation of tradition are important, important in their own right. Religion, as well as other ongoing human institutions, tends to lose sight of the original basis for assuring a given position. (It is human nature to remember only the conclusion, forgetting the details of all the pros and cons of the arguments.) There are conservative forces in religion, and yet, at the same time, organized religion must either meet the current needs of the people within certain limits or it will perish. In some respects, organized religion will be a dynamic force initiating changes. Historically, one of the situations in which organized religion has introduced change has been in supporting and "legitimizing" moral attitudes and practices for society. Some changes in social habits are much easier to make on a religious basis than on a legal basis. In most societies the two institutions are in such close agreement they often intermingle.

Rights of Society

The stand of organized Christianity, especially Roman Catholic, against birth control and abortion has been fulfilling the needs of the societies they serve. What are these needs of a society? The foremost function of a society is security. Security in a society depends on the people's ability to support themselves and to resist conquest by their neighbors. This latter security in large part depends on the size of the population: the number of soldiers that could be put on the battlefield. This was particularly true when men fought with spear and sword, and is not untrue today. Of course, this would not be true of nuclear warfare. Examples of societies with a need for large populations are the Middle Assyrian period, Israel before the Babylonian Captivity, and Hitler's Germany. This need was so great in ancient Israel that any attempt at population control was a sin. Abortion, masturbation, and coitus interruptus were forbidden. Himes, citing Jewish scholars, says the priests of that time distorted the meaning of the Talmud (Genesis 38:7-10) to support the prohibition against coitus interruptus (Onan) and masturbation (Er) in order to maintain good morals and preserve the race. The original meaning was that these two men refused to obey the law and perform the levirate marriage with their widowed sisters-in-law.

After the Babylonian Exile, the needs of the Jewish people changed, and there was a corresponding change in the moral law. Himes reports: (In this period) "the Jews settled down to a peaceful life.... By the time of Alexander the Great (330 B.C.), Palestine could no longer support all of its agricultural population. When the Jewish emigration and dispersion set in, large families were no longer regarded as a blessing.... Hence the race, adapting itself to the changed conditions, adopted new views and new practices. The old views and practices were protected and fortified by law and statute. The wording of the Mishna suggests that there was an old rigid law enjoining marriage and procreation under all circumstances and without any restrictions. The later stage of the law is satisfied with preservation of the race. After the birth of two children, the duty is fulfilled." After that time there was no other restriction against birth control. Himes states they also practiced embryotomy, a form of abortion in late gestation. It is not clear from Himes what, if any, restrictions were attached to this practice after 330 B.C. Before that time it was permissible to save the mother's life.

The above is an example of a society that changed its moral laws as its needs changed. Secure societies, such as ancient Egypt, Greece, and Rome, practiced birth control, abortion, and (in Greece and Rome) infanticide as a method of population control and a regulation of the responsibilities of motherhood. Himes further states with adequate evidence "that many primitive peoples thought in Malthusian terms long before Malthus" (the relationship between population growth and ability to provide food), and they used many means to reduce fertility, chief among which were coitus interruptus, abortion, and infanticide. In modern-day Japan abortion was legalized due to population pressure.

The alternative to population control in society with limited land and agriculture resources is the acquisition by conquest of new lands or emigration to other countries. Thus the New World, especially the United States, provided the outlet for European emigration for many centuries whereas wars, crusades, plagues, and colonialization had operated earlier—always the omnipresent wars. (The plague killed between one-fourth and one-half of the population of Europe in the fourteenth century.) Thus it would seem European societies (Christian societies) have, on the whole, needed to increase their populations because of these drastic events. There certainly has not been any need to limit the population until very recently.

The poor nation like a poor family needs a lot of people. Some oldsters used to say, "Children are money in the bank. The more you have, the more secure your old age." It is well recognized that as a country becomes more civilized and industrialized, its birthrate falls. Social security may have more to do with the increasing popularity of birth control in many parts of the world.

Today a large population and a high birthrate is seen as a liability rather than an asset from practically every point of view. Unless the per capita rate of economic growth is greater than the birthrate, a society cannot raise its standard of living. A major reason for this is the great reduction in the death rate of infants brought about by medical advances. Almost belatedly, concern is now being voiced not only about economic growth and standards of living, but about actual "livable" space on the globe.

Hence, today there would appear to be a clear need of societies in much of the world for a low birthrate, and the needs of a country would be expected to be reflected in its mores, including that of abortion.

What weight should we accord the needs of the state in deciding such a question?

Rights of the Fetus

With regard to the rights of the fetus, the Roman Catholic Church has taken an extreme position by placing the life of the unborn infant over that of its mother, even though she may have several other children. The Catholic Church's stand against abortion is consistent with its attitude toward contraception and toward the value of the fetus's life over that of the mother. However, the Church's stand against abortion also has a more important basis, a basis on which many Protestants and Jews concur: namely, the sacredness of human life. Catholics and some other sects, but not all, call abortion "murder." Yet the legal punishment for the crime of abortion is much less severe than that for murder. Few, if any, religious groups are urging that they be made the same. Abortion is certainly done with premeditation and forethought; therefore, if this were murder, it would be the worst degree of murder. Perhaps more important in pointing up the inconsistency of the abortion-is-murder attitude is the fact that the woman is usually not even considered to have committed a crime—only the abortionist. Yet she is certainly a principal in the act, and she pays for it. If a woman hired another man to kill her husband, and if her cooperation was necessary during the act, just how quickly do you suppose she would be arrested and found guilty?

The Biblical authority various religious denominations cite for their stand against abortion is Genesis 38:7-10 and Exodus 21:20-22, which is quoted below to show the content:

> "When a man strikes his slave, male or female, with a rod and the slave dies under his hand, he shall be punished. But if the salve survives a day or two, he is not to be punished; for the slave is his money.
>
> When men strive together, and hurt a woman with child, so that there is a miscarriage, and yet no harm follows, the one who hurt her shall be fined, according as the woman's husband shall lay upon him; and he shall pay as the judges determine."

The passage does not proffer a moral condemnation of abortion, but rather a law of restitution of property rights since the fetus's life is not of intrinsic value, but rather of meaningful value to the father.

Briefly, let us explore the question of when humanness of life begins. Some societies hold that life does not start until birth. Western income tax structures take the act of the first breath as a definition of life. If an infant is born dead, there is no tax deduction regardless of his size or birth weight; however, if the infant takes one breath and dies, that is, if he inflates his lungs, he is considered to have been alive and his parents are entitled to the full tax deduction.

Thirty-two weeks' gestation is usually taken as the point at which a fetus can survive outside the mother's body as a premature. There was a time when both English Common Law and the Roman Catholic Church took the first intrauterine movements of the infant as the beginning of life. (that would be in the fourth or fifth month of gestation.) Thus, the Church has not always considered abortion in the first three months to be against Canon Law, as is now the case.

It is also during the fourth month that the fetus psychologically becomes a "living person" to the mother. If a woman has a miscarriage in the first three months, there is usually less mourning reaction to the loss. However, if the miscarriage occurs after the fourth month, which is when the woman might feel the baby move, there is almost invariably a mourning period.

The heart of an unborn child does not begin to beat until the twelfth week after conception. There are also other significant changes that occur at about the twelfth week (end of the third month) of gestation, which greatly increase the technical difficulty and risk involved in an abortion.

Neither the intrauterine device nor the "morning-after pill" prevents fertilization; they prevent implantation of the fertilized ovum in the uterus. Some religious denominations approve of these methods, but the Roman Catholic Church does not.

The point of conception is the fusion of the ovum and sperm to form the genetic composition of the individual to be. Of course, there was a potential life every menstrual cycle. Certainly, each ovum and each sperm is very much alive and has potential for life. On the other extreme, one might say that an infant is not really human until he can do more than be startled, contented, or discontented; until he can smile in recognition, which does not begin until two to three months after birth.

So there is virtually an unbroken continuum of development to becoming human. Thus, deciding when an ovum—embryo—fetus—infant becomes human is primarily the business of philosophy and of religion, but which parts should be the business of law? Where should the rights of the unborn infant supersede the desires of the mother? Should the infant's rights extend to the act of sex itself? There was a time when religious law took precisely that stand: all sex was sinful except for intercourse for the sole purpose of procreation. Obviously the infant's right to life must begin somewhere. The rights of the embryo—fetus need to be weighed against the rights of the mother. The moral, the religious, and the legal scales need not be the same.

Rights of Women

What should be the sexual rights of women? Should any, some, or all women be legally and morally free to enjoy sex without fear of becoming pregnant? What about married women? Women on welfare? Single women? Women under sixteen or eighteen or twenty-one? Should legal sanctions be used to force a woman into the role of mother (1) To a child conceived or likely to be conceived by forceful rape? (2) To a child conceived in a moment or in a lifetime of indiscretion? (3) to a child conceived on the verge of divorce by a man she now loathes and hates? Should a woman be legally forced to carry the pregnancy of a man she does not love—or even hates?

Should a woman be legally forced to carry a pregnancy when the child is very likely to be born deformed? What about a child she hates, one she feels is a parasite inside of her? Should she be legally forced to carry a pregnancy when she knows the responsibility of raising him will disrupt her life and dash all her hopes and dreams for the kind of future she wants? Because of sexual indiscretion, or a tear in a condom, should a woman be legally forced to carry a pregnancy and deliver a child that she does not want or love and may actually hate? Should she not have a chance to rectify the error once she knows she is pregnant? Do we want to keep female sexual activity shackled to the obligations of motherhood with the iron chains of the law?

Laws to Enforce Morals

Will repeal or liberalization of the abortion law(s) change what you or I hold sacred? Is the legal question here similar to the legal question of the late sixteenth and the seventeenth centuries, when in various countries most professed belief as a protestant or a Catholic? Here law was used to force belief systems on the populace, and there were wars over it. Can we therefore in good consciousness and without self-righteousness use legal means to force our value system on others in so personal a matter?

A woman ought to have the legal right to decide whether or not to continue a pregnancy, at least up to twelve weeks of gestation, but probably not in the last two months, which is the time when the infant might be able to live outside of his mother. A woman who is pregnant because of irresponsible, carless, and immature sex, or because of honest miscalculation or accident (as well as carelessness in sex of a late middle-aged married couple), should have the right to decide whether or not to have the child. Once she knows that she is pregnant, she should have the right to rectify the error before being saddled with the full responsibility of raising a child to adulthood. Every child deserves to be wanted. As long as some children are wanted and others are not wanted or are even hated, men will never be created "equal."

We, as physicians, recognize the sacredness of human life and the fact that such belief is one of the cornerstones of civilization. Yet other considerations are also important: the woman's right to freedom of choice: the risk to herself and perhaps her family if her abortion is deemed criminal; the misery experienced by many unwanted children; the inhuman suffering of the unwed mother of whatever socio-economic class; and the injustice of criminal abortion based on money versus neglect of the underprivileged.

All of these considerations taken together certainly outweigh sentiment about the sacredness of a three- to six-month embryo-fetus, in our judgment.

PEG: It is worth emphasizing that the only really happy way to handle such situations is to not get pregnant, or not get a woman pregnant, in the first place. Plan. Plan your contraception. Every child has a right to be wanted. Know yourself; know your arousal pattern, and think. Do not get swept off your feet. Use your head. Decide. It is pretty much up to you to decide how far you are willing to go in petting, as in anything else. This is your decision, and I think, if you are considerate and consistent, you will have no serious trouble with it.

Chapter 15
Sexually Transmitted Disease

Sexually Transmitted Disease

Is vernereal disease still something we should be concerned about?

MARSHALL: I am afraid it is a serious problem. Venereal diseases, also called *sexually transmitted diseases (STDs)*, are contracted by one partner from another through sexual activity, sometimes involving little more than kissing or petting. The contact must be with an infected person; STDs do not appear spontaneously. STDs may be bacterial, viral, protozoal, fungal, or parasitic. Some present symptoms, but not always, and sometimes not at all. Many can cause serious harm to the body, and a few can lead to death. By their very nature, all are contagious, but all can be prevented by taking precautions. Most are curable, but at this time some are only treatable. Ignorance and indifference lead to too many new infections every year.

What about catching them from a washcloth, drinking glass, towel, or toilet seat?

Most, no. For example, HIV/AIDS requires an actual exchange of body fluids, not including saliva. However, the eggs of crabs are easily passed along through objects such as shared towels.

Are STDs very common?

The prevalence and rates vary considerably in different regions of the world, and they fluctuate both up and down over time. Statistics are difficult to gather accurately, as STDs are reported differently in different countries, sometimes not at all. It is safe to say that the vast majority of cases are not reported, even if they are treated.

STDs are known to affect people of all races and all socioeconomic classes, regardless of living conditions and hygiene. Adolescents tend to bear higher rates of STDs than their proportion of the population, probably owing to ignorance and less access to preventive measures. Even infants may suffer from STDs passed by their mothers during pregnancy or birth. STDs are more common than most people think, and the risks are greater than many want to believe.

Following are some of the most dangerous and/or common STDs:

Syphilis

Syphilis is a bacterial STD that causes sores to develop in the area of exposure, which is most likely the genitals and/or mouth. It tends to start as a painful red sore, which may not be detected if it is inside the vagina. Open sores tend to heal without scarring, often in 7-10 days, thus fooling the infected person into believing it has gone away. Other symptoms include fever, sore throat, headaches, and joint pain.

After the first stage with open sore(s), syphilis progresses to its second stage, which usually includes a faint rash over the entire body, plus a red rash that involves the palms of the hands and the soles of the feet. This, too, is likely to clear up without treatment, again fooling the patient.

The disease enters a third stage in which all the organs of the body are affected. However, the damage is so gradual that the effects may not be detected for ten, fifteen, or even twenty years. Cascading organ failures can lead to death and/or mental debility.

With even the slightest suspicion of syphilis infection, medical testing should confirm the diagnosis so treatment with antibiotics may begin.

Gonorrhea

Gonorrhea is a bacterial STD that may cause no initial symptoms, but most likely will be noticed first by a foul-smelling genital discharge and localized infections in both men and women, usually within 2-5 days, but possibly up to thirty days after exposure. Men may experience swollen testicles. Women may suffer from vaginal bleeding and pelvic inflammatory disease. Gonorrhea can infect both the mouth and genitals, then spread throughout the body, causing considerable damage. It can be cured with antibiotics.

Chlamydia

Chlamydia is considered to be the most prevalent bacterial STD in the USA. It is first noticed in women as itching around the vagina, a yellow and odorless discharge, pain during sex, and pain during frequent urination. Men will experience burning during urination, and a watery, milky-colored discharge from the penis. Within 1-3 weeks, more symptoms appear, including increased pain. It can be cured with antibiotics.

HIV/AIDS

Human Immunodeficiency Virus (HIV) is the most dangerous of the viral STDs. It progresses to *Acquired Immunodeficiency Syndrome (AIDS)*. AIDS is lethal. HIV is first noticed by fever, headache, rash, swollen lymph nodes, and fatigue. It progresses to diarrhea, weight loss, open sores, and late-stage infections. The dramatically weakened immune system resulting from AIDS often leads to other fatal diseases such as pneumonia, nervous system damage, and even cancer. Although research continues to seek a cure, treatment to limit the effects of the virus is available.

HPV/Genital Warts

Human Papilomavirus (HPV) is the most common of all kinds of STDs in the USA. It causes genital warts, though not every infected person develops them. Warts may appear on the penis, scrotum, vagina, anus, and surrounding areas. Warts generally appear about 1-3 months after infection. HPV is contagious, even without the presence of visible warts, but it is usually spread by direct contact with a wart. Some types of HPV also appear to increase the risk of cervical cancer. HPV is treatable, but not presently curable. A vaccine has been developed to aid in prevention.

Herpes

The *Herpes Simplex Virus (HSV)* is highly contagious, especially when coming in contact with open sores. *Genital herpes* shows symptoms only during an "attack" of the disease, but some people will never exhibit symptoms. They include pain and itching at the exposed site, small red blisters, and open sores. The blisters rupture and ooze blood and pus, during which painful urination, fever, headache, and muscle aches are common. The blisters eventually heal until the next attack. Herpes outbreaks at the mouth usually appear as blisters and "cold sores" on the lips and in the mouth. They are highly contagious during this stage, even with light kissing. Herpes is not contagious through casual contact with skin where no sores are present. People usually can prevent spreading herpes while still engaging in acts such as hugging, massage, and even mutual masturbation. No cure is available, but some treatments may reduce the severity of the attacks.

Crabs and Scabies

What are crabs?

PEG: *Crabs* and *scabies* and different species of *lice*. Crabs are found in the hairy regions of the body, usually in the pubic area. They are contracted via contact with an infected area, or from bedding, furniture, and clothing carrying *nits* (eggs). Scabies burrow into the skin and are known to cover wider areas of the body. While both of these parasites may be spread through sexual contact, non-sexual contact is just as risky, as is sharing space (e.g.: sitting on same sofa, using same hand towels, etc.) with an infected person. Shampoos, medicated soaps, and creams are available to kill these pests. Often, the entire family or all members of a household choose to undergo treatment at the same time.

Avoiding STDs

Abstinence is the most reliable method of avoiding STDs, followed by ensuring that sexual contact is only with a partner who is not infected. Unfortunately, some who carry STDs might not know it, while others might choose not to reveal it. Many in long-term relationships opt to undergo mutual testing for STDs before their relationship matures to intimate sexual activity.

Absent clear assurance that a sexual partner is free of STDs, precautions may be taken to reduce the chances of contracting them. Condoms, male and female, are highly effective if used properly. Spermicides are also known to kill many of the germs associated with STDs. Spermicides are most effective if used with condoms. Diaphragms, sponges, and caps inserted into the vagina, used with spemicide, can help protect the cervix from STDs.

Pregnant women with STDs should be sure to work with their medical team so steps can be taken to reduce the chances of transmitting STDs to their babies, and to reduce the chances of harm to the fetus.

The existence of STDs in the world should not scare people into avoiding the pursuit of a satisfying sex life. Just as we take precautions to prevent contracting all other kinds of diseases, from undergoing routine vaccinations to everyday casual handwashing, avoidance of STDs requires commonsense awareness and precautions.

Chapter 16
Marriage

Premarital Exam

Should a couple have a doctor's examination before they get married or begin a sexual relationship? If yes, what does it determine and how is it done?

PEG: Possibilities for the man include an examination of the genitalia and a blood test. This is just a screening for HIV, herpes, gonorrhea, syphilis, and other venereal diseases. The woman could benefit from a pelvic examination and a blood test. Examinations are a public health measure providing protection for the noninfected person and unborn children.

This is also an excellent time for you to bring up any marital-oriented questions you may wish to ask your physician. I usually discussed douching, "honeymoon cystitis," and "marriage rules and regulations" with my patients.

Douching

Douching is just washing out the vagina with plain water or water plus some additive. It is not necessary from a health standpoint, since the vagina is fully capable of cleansing itself with its discharge; however, some women feel more feminine by doing this. Actually, all odors connected with intercourse can be adequately taken care of by a regular bath.

Honeymoon Cystitis

Honeymoon Cystitis is an infection of the bladder. It produces symptoms of painful urination, increased frequency of urination, increased urgency to urinate, and sometimes a bloody urine. The infection should be treated promptly by a physician.

Rules and Regulations of Marriage

Rules and regulations of marriage are a number of rather commonsense concepts that should be brought to the attention of proposed newlyweds. For example:

1. Set up some ground rules ahead of time for occasions when you have disagreements: (a) Communicate your hurt rather than your anger or resentment at being hurt. You have an obligation by just being in love to communicate your hurt. (b) Do not shout at each other; this alone will keep the argument on a certain level. Volume does not win. (c) Settle the dispute as quickly as possible. Resentment unexpressed grows much more often than it fades. (d) Do not take your troubles to anyone other than a professional. Do not attempt to seek advice at work or from acquaintances; it just is not there. (e) Do not leave the house angry and, better yet, never go to bed angry.

2. Do not fall into the habit of making your partner the brunt of jokes. Some couples have this down to a fine art; much hostility is vented in a situation where the partner feels defenseless unless willing to make a scene. If you must make fun, do it positively: "He's the most considerate... the best planner and manager," etc., and let the crowd wonder what the grain of truth is in that.

3. Do not do bathroom chores while your mate is using the bathroom for other purposes. Early in a relationship, this will enhance the romantic aspect of your marriage. After you have been married for a while, this may not be an im-

portant factor, although privacy can remain a significant need in many people.

4. Never in a state of pique make any derogatory remark about your partner's sexual attractiveness or sexual adequacy. This is much too severe and should never be played with. Someone else may tell you you are fat and unattractive, but you cannot take it from the person you love. This makes a "hurt" that may never completely heal, no matter how many positive experiences and remarks are piled upon it. Part of loving is being exceptionally vulnerable to a person's criticism and disapproval, especially in the sexual area. This vulnerability to each other should be acknowledged and all necessary precautions taken to avoid hurting the one you love.

Frequency of Intercourse in Marriage

How often do fully involved couples have intercourse on the average? What is the frequency for the first years of married life?

MARSHALL: It will vary with age. This category varies less with socio-economic class than other categories do. Kinsey reports an average of 3.9 times a week for 16- to 20-year-olds, falling to 2.9 for the 25- to 30-year-olds. The average continues to decrease with age. However, there is great variation. Some normal and healthy couples have intercourse once a month, and others that are sexually athletic have it two to three times a day. Again, frequency of intercourse should be discussed openly, fully, and freely between the marriage partners. One's feelings about the frequency of intercourse, like one's views and value system, should be communicated and respected. By age 41 to 45 the frequency rate has dropped to about 1.5 times per week.

Sexual Compatibility

How long does it take for a couple to become sexually compatible?

MARSHALL: I take that to mean both the man and woman are content with their giving and receiving of sexual gratification. In part this will depend on what their expectations are. Some individuals and couples feel they ought to achieve orgasm at about the same time. This is unrealistic. Masters and Johnson have shown this rarely happens, even with the subjects they studied.

Other people believe sexual compatibility means that the woman must have an orgasm every time. This, too, is unrealistic, because distractions also occur during intercourse in married life; take a baby's cry, for instance. Mild fatigue may be a hindrance to orgasm. There is nothing wrong if a woman does not get that excited every time. Remember, too, that intercourse ends when the man loses his erection, shortly after his orgasm. If the woman is not close to orgasm at that time, she will not reach it without additional stimulation, perhaps digitally or orally. Another alternative would be to engage in sex play for several minutes until the man has another erection. There is great individual variation here, too. A few men will not lose their erection when they ejaculate. Others have a refractory period of up to 30 to 40 minutes. The time interval increases with age. If the woman achieves orgasm first, the man may go on and reach it several minutes later. Some women on occasion may have two or three orgasms in one act of intercourse while their partner has only one. How rapidly a couple achieves realistic, mutual, sexual satisfaction depends primarily on communication. Chiefly it is communication (and elimination) of distracting elements in the environment or in the interaction of sexplay and the communication of the state of readiness of the woman. Some couples cannot communicate and never achieve it. The woman may think that she is frigid. Other couples, by being considerate of each other, communicating rather freely, and learning their own sexual responses and that of their partner, achieve it rather quickly.

"Cooling" with Time

I have heard that marriages "cool" after a few years. Is this true? I mean, does the wife really become less attractive to her husband in both the physical and emotional senses of love?

PEG: I think this depends on what foundation the relationship has and what is going on in it. I think it depends on what the people are looking for, how much they are willing to give, how completely of themselves they can give, how considerate and interested they are in the other person. There is not any rule that you can only have fun for the first few years. Your relationship, your marriage, just like anything else, is what you make it. If you are willing to invest yourself in your spouse and in your marriage, you will do well. If you are just sitting back waiting to be given to, you are very likely to have some cooling.

MARSHALL: I think that over the years there is a natural tendency for married couples to fall into a routine and to take each other for granted; so there is a tendency for marriages to cool. But when (and if) you notice this, either of you can reintroduce some magic; invest something. The relationship need not cool. Love is based on the feeling that your mate is extra special, so reintroduce part of that pedestal you had your spouse on. A night out once a week can do wonders. Just have fun together, just the two of you. If you find you are only going out with another couple, beware; it is an early sign of boredom. Going out together is well worth the price of baby-sitters and even a meal away from home. You do not need those few dollars or a new washing machine that badly. Spice can be added at home in little things, too—an extra kiss or pat, his favorite food, candlelight, even for the whole family, because children get enjoyment out of it. And do not forget the sexual area itself. Remember that at least once in a while a woman should initiate intercourse. It is one way of reassuring a husband that you love him and enjoy sex and are not just going along. And put some variation in it, especially in foreplay. You may spend hours planning and preparing a meal for your husband or wife, yet let yourself exist on the same sexual diet of mashed potatoes or warmed-over beans for years.

Extramarital Affairs

PEG: There is a major distinction between a marriage that has cooled and one in which there is an extramarital affair. The basic reason people remain faithful to one another is their awareness of how deeply not doing so would hurt their mates.

MARSHALL: the converse is also true. Extramarital affairs occur when the spouse either does not care or encourages the affair, openly, covertly, or ambivalently. Sexual difficulties are the most common cause for one partner encouraging the other to have sex with someone else.

For example, common misconceptions about sex place the primary responsibility for sexual gratification of both partners on the man, with the concept that a woman only has to make herself available and the man does it all. If the couple accept this false standard, and if the woman is non-orgasmic, it is not uncommon for her to experiment to see if another man is better. Actually, her husband may encourage it, either as a check on his own adequacy or as a relief of responsibility. The non-orgasmic wife may also push her husband to another woman by making him feel totally inadequate as a man, either because he is inadequate to bring her to orgasm, or because she is inadequate as a woman.

PEG: Of course, the same principles apply when the man has sexual difficulties. Often the wife feels inadequate as a woman because she cannot stimulate him "in the right way."

Intercourse and Pregnancy

How long before delivery is it that you can have intercourse?

PEG: Except in unusual cases, intercourse until the last six weeks before delivery is considered safe. After that, seek the advice of your obstetrician.

How long after delivery before you can have intercourse?

PEG: This will vary with how uncomfortable it would be for the woman. After delivery the area around the vagina might have sutures in it, and, until healing takes place, it can be painful with pressure and movement. A standard procedure is to abstain for six weeks after the delivery.

Effects of Aging in Men

Does male potency decline with age, or does it depend completely on psychological factors?

MARSHALL: I have seen one report including men up to age 96 enjoying sexual intercourse. In this particular geriatric group, there was a couple of about 76 who had stopped because they did not think their children would approve. Kinsey reports that men age 56 to 60 are having intercourse about once a week and that 70 percent of men aged 66 to 70 are still having some intercourse. The number of sperm per ejaculation does drop markedly with old age. Masters and Johnson's second book has greatly expanded knowledge in this area. They indicate that the greatest detriment to sexual performance in older age groups is the popular belief there will come a time, due to aging, when ability to perform will be lost. For example, there only remains for the man to experience some small impairment in functioning on one occasion, which he would overlook if younger, to cause him to become worried and to begin to wonder about his ability to achieve an erection during the act of intercourse, rather than just giving of himself, and he cannot perform. This situation snowballs until he is convinced he is too old. Masters and Johnson have shown that in the aging process there is a decrease in sex drive, delayed erective reaction, and a decrease in the force of ejaculation. They state that for both male and female the most important factor in maintaining sexual functioning in old age is consistency of sexual functioning.

Erectile Dysfunction

Erectile Dysfunction (ED) refers to difficulty achieving and/or maintaining an erection. The best treatment or combination of treatments should be determined in consultation with a physician and/or therapist, and will depend on the cause. Most men normally experience gradual decreases in erectile function with aging, which can also be treated. Loss of erectile capability makes intercourse difficult, but does not preclude mutually satisfying sexual activity, nor is an erection required to achieve ejaculation.

While some erectile difficulties may be caused by psychological factors, even those with physical bases have a psychological effect on both the man and his partner. Consulting with a sex therapist may prove to be beneficial to the relationship.

The common treatment is use of oral medications that block an enzyme in the body so that, when combined with sexual stimulation, they will help blood flow into the penis. The popular three are tadalafil (Cialis in the USA), vardenafil (Levitra in the USA), and sildenafil (Viagra in the USA). In most countries these are available with a physician's prescription. Patients should be careful to monitor for side effects, especially when the effects are unfamiliar.

Other treatments include "the penis pump," a mechanical device; penile implants, which are prostheses of varying types; surgery to correct blood-flow problems or damaged tissue; and many "natural remedies" whose effectiveness usually is not well documented, but which may prove effective if only for psychological reasons.

Other forms of treatment are available in some parts of the world, but not approved in others. Others are still being researched and/or tested. These include dopamine stimulators; various creams, injections, and suppositories; drugs that act through the central nervous system; and gene therapy.

Testicle Exam

Adolescent boys and men should conduct monthly testicle self-exams beginning by the age of 14 and continuing for life. Exams can lead to early discovery of several kinds of possible problems, but their greatest value is for early detection of testicular cancer. This is one of the most common cancers in men, especially those younger than age 35. It is important for young adolescents to do these exams routinely so you are familiar with this important area of your body. Then you will be able to notice small changes right away, which is when treatment carries a very high cure rate.

Early treatment of cancer can help protect your reproductive capability. Early treatment of a *sexually transmitted disease (STD)* can help protect your own health as well as your partner's. Men do not have to be sexually active to develop testicle problems. Cancer is not caused by masturbation or sex with a partner.

These exams are best performed after a warm bath or shower when the scrotum is relaxed. Using a mirror makes it easier to spot swelling of the scrotal skin. Each testicle should be checked with both hands, gently rolled between thumbs and fingers. You should not feel pain. Do not be concerned about one testicle being slightly larger than the other.

Notice the normal feel of the epididymis, the soft tubelike structure behind the testicle for collecting and carrying sperm. You are looking for lumps (most likely on the sides or fronts), unusual enlargement or shrinkage of a testicle, a feeling of heaviness in the scrotum, a dull ache in the area, the presence of fluid in the scrotum, or anything significantly different from previous exams.

When in doubt, check it out. Do not delay seeing a physician. You may first become aware of a problem when your partner notices a change. Do not dismiss these observations just because you detect nothing obvious. If you are a young teen feeling embarrassed about expressing concerns to your parents, you could ask someone you trust to help you broach the subject, or see the doctor yourself and pay for it. However you seek medical attention, remember that protecting your health is one of the most important responsibilities of being a man.

Effects of Aging in Women

Does menopause do anything to a woman's ability to have intercourse?

Menopause, per se, need not interfere in any way with normal sexual functioning. As a result of aging, it may take somewhat longer for the vagina to lubricate, and orgasms may not be as intense physically as they were at a younger age, but intercourse will remain just as fulfilling, pleasurable, and satisfying psychologically as it always was. Some women may need sex hormone replacement following menopause to keep the vaginal tissues in a satisfactory physiologic state for intercourse, but that may carry risks that should be discussed with your physician.

PEG: Physically, after menopause the hormonal shifts that regularly went on no longer take place; there are no menstrual cycles. Actually, sexual excitement, as we have pointed out before, is mainly psychological, so reaching the menopause would not necessarily mean that the woman would no longer be able to enjoy sexual intercourse. The frequencies of marital intercourse for married women living with their husbands is exactly the same as that for married men.

Breast Exam

How do you do a self-examination of the breasts for cancer?

Self-examination of the breasts should be done at least once a month. You are feeling for lumps. Feel with the flat of your hand using your right hand on your left breast and vice versa, when you are in an upright position and when you are flat in bed. Your breasts will vary in their consistency during your menstrual cycle. Just prior to the menstrual period they might feel quite lumpy or nodular, but this will disappear after the period. You need to know what is normal for you so that you will be more likely to spot an unusual lump. If you do find one, you should have it checked by a doctor. Every woman should also have a Pap smear at intervals recommended by her physician.

Chapter 17
Parenting and Child Sexual Development

Early Childhood

In *Paradise Lost*, Milton has Satan say that the mind can make a heaven of hell, or a hell of heaven. When looking at the attitudes that various societies have held toward sex, one can readily see the truth of the statement.

Of all things that parents can teach children in regard to sex, the most important will be the attitude toward sex and sexual functions, which more than any other single factor will determine whether as adults they can achieve sexual satisfaction and fulfillment, or whether sex will always be something bad, tainted, dirty; something never to be talked about even to one's spouse.

The gender of the child, even as early as three months of age, influences the way parents respond to that child. Parents tend to talk to their girl infants much more than to their boy infants; however, they reward crying, thereby rewarding assertiveness in baby boys to a much greater extent than in baby girls. Undoubtedly many other parental attitudes determined by the sex of the child affect his or her future development.

Many parents have been self-conscious and embarrassed about answering a child's questions about sex, which somehow seems rather strange. Parents certainly know more about sex, and sexual questions can be answered more logically than "What makes the stars twinkle?" or "What is war, and why do people kill each other?" Yet PTA groups and other organizations are devoted to helping parents explain sex to children or explaining it for them, while there is apparently less difficulty in explaining war to children.

Age Two to Six

A child of age two or three first becomes aware that adults and humans are divided into two sexes. Prior to that time, the child has been differentiating animate objects from inanimate objects and people from other animals. Indeed, there are greater similarities between male and female humans than between humans and other animals, and it is with this level of discrimination that the child has been preoccupied prior to the age of two.

This awareness of the complete set being comprised of only two sexes has been preceded by people using the words as they point out boys and girls, men and women, etc. Unless people having been saying what he or she is, the child almost invariably asks, "Am I a boy or a girl?" Parents have little difficulty explaining this and may go on to point out that girls grow up to be women and boys grow up to be men.

Perhaps the first genital question becomes, "Daddy, why do girls sit down to go to the potty and why do boys stand up?" This question, like all other sexual questions, should be answered as openly and honestly and as simply as the question is asked. "Boys and men have a penis and so they can sort of aim their water or urine, but girls and women don't, so they have to sit down."

Consider the significance to the child of the above "fact." Did you ever tell a three-year-old child that he had anything that somebody else did not have or that somebody else had something that she did not have? Consider bringing home a present for one child and not bringing one for a three- or four-year-old. Children of this age invariably want what the other child has. If the child obtains the item, the satisfaction is only momentary. This is also the age of exploration of the body and the body's capabilities. The pride in being able to turn a somersault or climb a tree is tremendous. This testing of body capability extends to the functions of elimination.

Almost invariably the boys try to urinate sitting down, which presents no difficulty, and the girls try to urinate standing up, perhaps several times. In psychoanalytic theory this total situation leads into what has been called "penis envy" in little girls, which usually is temporary. However, if a girl gets "hung up" on it somehow (fixated), there may be derivatives which carry over into adult life.

It is also at about this age that the child will ask, "What does married mean?" This concept may arise from the awareness that other children refer to their parents as "Mommy" and "Daddy" and that these are generic terms and not proper names, or from noticing differences among family structures including single parents, a parent who lives separately or is married to another, and calling proximate parent figures by other labels to distinguish a somewhat different relationship. The married question usually does not produce the concern and anxiety in parents that more sexual kinds of questions do. It is answered as, "When a man and woman love each other and want to live together always and have a family, they usually get married. They may have babies, little boys and little girls." One should not be concerned about all the exceptions in the basic pattern at this point; if the question is answered openly and without embarrassment when the child confronts one of the variations, such as a playmate with only one parent, he will ask and will be ready for the information. The next logical question is, "Where do the babies come from?" This question may be immediate, but will usually occur somewhere between half an hour and six months later. The question may arise from a sequence such as "Is Grandma really your mother? Does everybody have a mother and daddy? Why?" It may also come up in the following way: "Daddy, how old am I? How old are you?" with some concept and awareness of quantity comes the invariable question, "Where was I before I started adding years?" or "Where was I before I was born?" The answer: "You were inside mother, right up under her heart. Mother carried you around inside of her until you were ready to come out."

I prefer the phrase "in her abdomen" or "under mother's heart" to "tummy," thus avoiding confusion with "stomach." This may be a small point. I am sure that many thousands of children are told that they grow inside mother's "tummy" and have no difficulty from this. However, in my work as a child psychiatrist, I have seen many kinds of problems which involve the use of the word "tummy." For example, if a child is told perhaps weeks or months apart that he grows from a seed that daddy puts in mother's tummy, that things that he eats go into his tummy, and that orange trees grow from orange seeds, then he would have to conclude from a strictly logical basis that if he eats an orange seed, he will have an orange tree growing in his tummy. This information, or misinformation, or misinterpretation of the information leads the child into fantasies of becoming pregnant by taking things in the mouth. This unconscious fantasy appears to be very common among male homosexuals. The fantasy is also involved in cases of anorexia nervosa (nervous loss of appetite), a severe emotional illness which is most often found in girls near the time of puberty. Therefore, I recommend that in explaining where the baby grows, care is taken to separate the stomach from the uterus, even if just to say in a separate special place where babies grow. Give the child time to mull this information over and, in moments or weeks, he will ask, "How do babies get out of their mothers?" "Women have a little opening between their legs that boys and men don't have. This is called the vagina. When the baby is ready to come out, this opens up and lets the baby come out. Animals make easy comparisons for children exposed to pets giving birth, or for those living in breeding environments such as farms. Nearly all environments will present occasional opportunities to point out how an obviously pregnant woman means she is growing her very own baby, which will be born soon. Again this takes the mystery out of it. Save the labor pains, etc., until the child asks more about the process or at least until he or she is at the prepuberty age.

Another rather common misconception which gets covered over by time and may (rarely) cause unhappiness in later life is the concept that babies are born via the rectum and anus; hence, the phrase "an opening that boys don't have." Aside from aesthetics, this is the reason delivery should not be explained via analogy to bowel movements.

Usually closely associated in time with the question of how babies are born is the question, "How do babies get started?" or "Where was I before I was inside Mother?" "When two people are in love and want children, the man puts part of himself—sort of half a human seed—inside the mother's opening, her vagina. That half seed finds a half seed which is part of the mother, and a whole seed is made that begins to grow in mother's uterus." One should mention both "human" and "half" in connection with the seed (or egg, if that word is personally preferable to seed). In either event, it should be clear one is using an analogy, and it has little to do with apple seeds, grapefruit seeds, or breakfast eggs.

"How does a daddy put the half seed in a mommy's vagina?" "With his penis. The penis is used to urinate with (pass your water), and when boys become men it can also be used to put the seed in mothers' vaginas."

"Daddy, show me a half a human seed."

"I can't do that; they are inside my body and only come out when two people are making love. That's the way we are (or that's just the way God made us)."

As stated before, if the child can formulate the question, he is ready for an answer. He should be given an answer rather than ever being told something, such as "You're too young to know," or "We'll talk about that when you're older." With this type of non-answer the child understands "There are some things my parents don't want me to know." Usually he will never ask that parent another sex question. At times he enlarges the scope of the

"I am not supposed to know" to include the other parent (frequently) and to all learning in general, i.e., schoolwork (infrequently). If, indeed, the child is too young to know, he will really not believe the answer. For example, if a two-year-old does happen to ask, "Where do babies come from?" and is told that they grow inside mother, he usually will not believe it. He will think that babies come from the store, just like everything else that is brought into the house comes from the store. The only difference is that this kind of store, as opposed to the grocery store or the hardware, may be called a hospital. No harm is done by an honest answer which the child is not ready for or cannot understand. Harm can be done by too large or involved an answer. If the child changes the subject or becomes disinterested, drop the subject; that is enough for the time being.

Concepts of Death

It is at age three to six that children can conceptualize such questions as "Where was I before I got born?" And paralleling the questions of sex and life are those about life and death. We know less about death than sex, but most parents have little difficulty with this topic. The specific answers are chiefly dependent upon one's religious beliefs. Often interest in the subject will be triggered by the death of someone known to the child, or by the death of a pet or other animal. Some children are quick to enlarge the concept of mortality from animals to humans, while others may have an interval before coming to that realization.

Sexual Feelings

The forerunners to feelings of sexual arousal and excitement, those feelings in the adult that are attendant to sex play, begin before one year of age with the pleasurable "tickle game." Tickling has several things in common with foreplay. In both instances the other person must be familiar and trusted. A stranger or someone disliked cannot elicit the response. Both involve touch which is moderately light and moving. By age three to four, the sexual feelings are frequently attached to words and, since the differences between boys and girls are most poignant in the bathroom, to words of elimination.

Masturbation

Children also produce the feeling by self-stimulation, such as jumping up and down, especially astride an object, and a little later by manual stimulation of their genitals—masturbation. Up to the time of masturbation, the child has used thumb sucking (or one of its variants) as the mode of pleasurable self-stimulation. Thumb sucking produces feelings of satisfaction, contentment, and security; not the nigh, giddy excitement of masturbation. (Dentists are generally agreed that thumb sucking which persists after the eruption of the permanent teeth will cause malocclusion.) Self-stimulation in older children and adults includes daydreaming. Many daydreams are sexually exciting, but essentially any emotion can be produced by the thoughts of a daydream. The various forms of self-stimulation tend to occur when the individual is bored, has nothing to do, or is in a state between sleep and wakefulness. The period just before falling asleep is the most common time for self-stimulation activity.

The most detrimental effect of masturbation is generally the guilt that parents (and then the children) may attach to the act. In girls there is also some danger of a bladder infection with prolonged masturbation, especially if the genital area is not kept clean. Girls have a relatively short urethra (tube leading from the bladder to the outside), so prolonged rubbing may introduce bacteria. Women may also get a bladder infection with frequent intercourse (cystitis). Young girls should be taught to wipe themselves away from the genitals and not the reverse, even though it may seem less natural.

Parents are usually justifiably concerned with the social aspects of masturbation, and the best way to handle this is to teach the child the distinction between public and private behavior. Since children learn this concept quickly, it actually may be taught at about age two-and-a-half in regard to thumbsucking. Saying something like, "Thumbsucking is all right when you are about to go to sleep or when you are alone and by yourself, but it is not something that you do out in front of other people." Consequently, when the masturbation becomes prominent, the same attitude can readily be taken. As the child becomes an adult, he or she does not have to unlearn any attitudes toward pleasure from the genital area. He or she already knows that it is something intimate, something done in private, and that there is nothing intrinsically wrong with it, nothing to be ashamed of, but that he or she should control expressions of the accompanying feelings.

Sexual excitement, like any other feelings, are sensations that we want the child to experience in degree so he or she can learn to control their expression without being swept away by their strength. We hope to avoid a child being carried away beyond his or her ability to reason and to act in one's own best interest.

Sexual Roles

Another basic determinant of sexual feelings in childhood is that of sex in the largest sense of the word—that is, the sexual roles. Between ages three and four there is a marked growth in awareness of sexual roles. All societies assign sexual roles to varying degrees. Even if that were not so, children of this age would ascribe sexual roles to observed differences in behavior such as the division of labor between parents. They learn the rules and the taboos in choosing a marriage partner, which is generally preferable. In our society, examples of rule include that the partner be of the opposite sex, of about the same age, and from outside the family. In their headlong rush to grow up, and knowing that they and one of their parents are of the same sex, they wish to emulate or identify with this parent. This identification may apply to bathroom habits and common activities around the home. In all things and in all ways, the child wishes to be really grown up now, to be like the identified parent. The child observes behavior patterns of the parent and may doggedly insist on doing the same things in the same order. This behavior has actually begun earlier, about age one-and-a-half, and it frequently begins in the bathroom. The child may demand that the bathroom door be closed, but it makes no difference who is inside or outside the bathroom. Children will play at doing yard work or preparing a meal. (They may actually "help," although their helping may make more work for the adult. Parents should appreciate these opportunities to influence their children's burgeoning attitudes toward work.) However, children are also aware that part of the role of being a parent is the little understood function of making babies with the parent of the opposite sex. They wish to be grown up in this way, also. Consequently, in almost all children there is the wish to make a baby in an emulation of the parent of the same sex. The baby is obviously to be made with the parent of the opposite sex, and here all kinds of thoughts and feelings may come in. Many of the psychological difficulties that may ensure later on can be avoided by some judicious handling.

Almost all children who feel free to talk with their parents say something about marrying the parent of the opposite sex and making or having a baby with them. This situation is best handled by, "That's okay, but children just don't marry their parents. Boys and girls marry somebody about their own age. When you are grown up and ready to get married, you can find somebody you would like to marry." And then as an afterthought, "But I guess it's sort of fun thinking about it anyhow, huh? That's okay, too." Children have and will have these daydreams, regardless of what adults might say. As these daydreams continue, the child is thrown into a daydream rivalry with his parent of the same sex. "If it weren't for daddy, I bet I could make a baby with mother." At the same time, the child loves both parents. The minds of people are such that this quasi-conflict between the love of the real relationship and the rivalry of the daydream makes a child anticipate the parent of the same sex having the same thoughts toward him or her. Furthermore, because of these thoughts, the child deserves to have done to him or her what was daydreamed being done to the parent—that is, getting rid of the rival. The child imagines and embellishes how he or she might be gotten rid of. Part of the thought of physical retribution from the parent soon becomes unconscious, but comes to consciousness again in the fear of bodily injury, fear of the dark, and the nightmares of the four- to six-year-old. Such fears are almost universal at this age, even in children who previously had been fearless.

In addition to what the parent might say to the child, the most helpful thing is for the parent of the same sex to say something such as "I know you love your mommy; that's good. I also know you sometimes think of marrying her and that's okay, too. You can't marry anyone till you grow up, but it's all right to think about it. I don't care; I still love you." It is surprising how this sort of statement can greatly reduce or eliminate chronic fears of nightmares. (Note: Other common causes of nightmares are sibling rivalry and the death of someone in the family or a loved pet.)

At the same time, the parent of the opposite sex should avoid any interaction with the child which is sexually stimulating, especially actions that produce an emotion of heightened silliness or giddiness. This is not to say the child should not ever have feelings of sexual excitement with the parent of the opposite sex between the ages of four to six; far from it. Do not let the child get carried away, and do not do it too frequently. A child may be quite sexually stimulated by the parent of the opposite sex giving him or her a bath. The child will act in a hyperactive, silly, giddy fashion, and at this point the parent may encourage the youngster to wash his or her own private areas, or let the parent of the same sex give future baths. Also bed-sharing with the parent of the opposite sex should be strictly avoided.

One should also bear in mind that children, up until this time in their lives, regardless of whatever they have been able to conceptualize, have been ready to attempt to perform with their bodies. In short, their physical growth and development have kept ahead of their mental growth and development. Making babies is the first area in which they can roughly conceptualize but cannot attempt, and for them, this is because they do not know enough about how to do it.

Sexual Curiosity

This ignorance gives rise to an extremely heightened curiosity in general and sexual curiosity in particular. Children's curiosity takes many forms, from an inquisitiveness and a probing intrusiveness to explorations of all kinds. At one time, children may recall that they only thought there was one kind of genitals; then they learned that there were two (male and female). They may ask their parents and be told there are only two and then encounter two males, only one of whom is circumcised, and they think maybe there are three types. "How many more types are there?" This uncertainty results in the inclination to examine and show genitals. After this peak of sexual curiosity, comes the recognition that their knowledge is utterly inadequate. Children have also been told that they will grow up to be mommies and daddies, and, when they grow up, they can perform adequately. All this, plus the love and simultaneous rivalry with the parent of the same sex, leads around age seven to a resignation and to a diminution of interest in sexual activity.

Age Eight to Ten

By age eight, children begin using sex words and telling sex jokes. By age nine, there is some sex swearing, some sex poems, and interest in sexual images. Again, some of this activity is just to stimulate sexual feelings in themselves and friends. But much of it is testing to see what reactions friends, adults, and especially parents will have to hearing the words. The words may also be used to express hostility. The parent's response should be based on the child's emotion. "You can get your anger out better than that." Or if the child is trying to shock, "Okay, so you have learned some new words and are playing with them, but how about turning them off for a while? I'm tired of them." If the child's emotion is quite excited, it might be ignored or, if it seems he or she is looking for a response, "Sounds like your feelings are about to run away with you; better tone it down."

There is also a new round of sex questions at around age ten. Parents will have to supply more detailed information to such questions as, "How does the baby really get out?" "Hospitals are places where operations occur. Does the baby come out with an operation? Is mother cut open? Does it hurt to have a baby? How much does the baby cost?" These questions should be answered honestly and fully. Much more information can be volunteered. Again, if the child becomes restless or inattentive, he or she has had enough for the time being.

Interest in Sexual Materials

The child's interest in sexual images and stories usually begins with less provocative material that is easily accessible, then may progress to seeking out more explicit material, maybe even pornography (material specifically intended only to arouse sexual feelings). Your major clue to dealing with your child will be his or her emotion, just as it was in regard to the use of sex words. In addition, you can take some clues from the material itself. Often your best response is no response other than nonverbally acknowledging you know he or she is looking at such images or reading such stories and they are approved. If you notice your child curious about ads for menstrual aids, it is time for a discussion on menstruation. If he or she is using reference materials, it is time for more sex discussions and your assistance in helping to obtain the proper educational books. Again, your attitude of "It's all right to know" is important. While every child who is not inhibited will look at pornography, very few actively seek it out and make a habit of looking at it. An active search for pornography occurring over several months would be indicative of something amiss emotionally in the child, and that needs attention.

If you notice your child with pornographic material, do not overreact; say something such as "You seem a little ashamed that I saw you with those pictures. You ought to know there are such pictures and to some people that's all sex means. When they portray sex, it's without love, without consideration of the other person. They imply that the only thing that's important is the genitals, not who the other person is, or what they mean to each other. That's why I don't like them; they show sex as separate from love." You may want to expand on this by one or two sentences (not too much). But a statement that ties into the basis of his or her value system—for example, religion or future maximum happiness—might be helpful.

Menstrual Education

BE SURE, ABSOLUTELY SURE, you have explained to your daughters the process of menstruation before it happens to them. Without advance knowledge of its significance, girls conclude they are injured or diseased and are quite fearful. But the reaction does not stop there, and they also go on to consider why and how it happened to them. They were bad; they masturbated; they had sexual thoughts, etc. The damage of these conjectures can probably never be wholly undone.

It is difficult to know the age at which a girl will begin to menstruate. A mother might take into account the age at which she and her mother-in-law began to menstruate. She should bear in mind that the age range from nine to fifteen is considered normal, and that on the average girls are menstruating at a younger age with each succeeding generation, presumably due to better nutrition and general health. The girl should be told that menstruation is part of growing up just like breast development and new hair growth. Menstruation is blood and fluids from inside her uterus; blood that was there to nourish a baby if one of her ova (eggs) was fertilized. Since it was not needed, the blood was discharged, and the cycle will repeat itself. All women menstruate about once a month, but when a girl first starts, her periods are very irregular. Menstruation is nothing to be ashamed of; it is just a private thing. When a girl first notices she is menstruating she should go to her mother, or, if away from home, to the teacher or a girlfriend's mother so that they will show her how to take care of herself. Most importantly, aside from knowledge of the phenomenon itself, is the attitude toward menstruation which is conveyed to the child. Menstruation is a normal female function and a sign of maturity and fertility rather than the curse of womankind. To a large extent a girl's attitude toward being a woman will be determined by her attitude toward her menses, and she will be reminded of it on the average of four to five days out of every twenty-eight.

Boys who show curiosity and a burgeoning awareness of the concept of menstruation deserve honest explanations, as well. It should not be treated as some mysterious secret they are not allowed to know. It should also be emphasized that most girls and women generally consider it a private matter, not an appropriate subject for immature teasing or jokes.

Nocturnal Emissions

Likewise, boys should be told of nocturnal emissions before they occur. The explanation should be clear and frank: "Nocturnal emissions are the discharges of semen from your penis during sleep, usually accompanied by a sexual dream. This is normal. The emissions (or "wet dreams") are part of growing to manhood, just as the development of a beard is. The semen contains sperm (half seed) and secretions of other sexual glands. This means you are now probably capable of fathering children. Since you had an excess of semen which was not discharged by intercourse or masturbation, your body just gets rid of it. There is nothing to worry about. Just change your pajamas and sheets as necessary, put them with the other dirty clothes, and go back to bed. No special steps are necessary in the laundry process." Knowledge of the laundry process may be a relief to him; it means there is no need for him to tell his mother of the nocturnal emission.

It is also important to mention that with masturbation there may not be the accumulation of semen and hence no nocturnal emission. All boys masturbate and, having been told nocturnal emissions are normal, fear something is wrong if they are no longer having the emissions. Most commonly they fear they might be sterile, and thus spend a good deal of energy worrying. The fantasies may be much more elaborate. As the boy continues to masturbate (for no boy stops, even with this worry) feelings of guilt and inadequacy get linked with those of sexuality, which may cause significant problems in later life.

Of course, it is also necessary to tell children about the physiology of the other sex. This should be done after they know about the physiology of their own sex. For the boy, it is best to start by noting in the girl the obvious changes, such as breast development and distribution of body fat before explaining menstruation. Likewise, with a girl, talk about the boy's mustache development and increased musculature, then go into nocturnal emissions and erections.

Normal Homosexual Attachments

In boys and girls the period of preadolescence and early adolescence is of crucial significance in regard to emotional development. For about two years prior to puberty, there is a period of a very intimate, confidential relationship with a peer of the same sex. This deep friendship is crucial for the ability to form deep, lasting relationships with both men and women in later life. Boys or girls having such a relationship share many secrets, some of which are sexual. With approaching adolescence, sexual matters are more and more important, and quite frequently overt homosexual experiences may take place between the pair. This may be mutual masturbation or even oral sex. These acts are no more indicative of a later homosexual orientation than sexual explorations at age five are indicative of promiscuity as an adult, and, if they do occur again, no great harm will be done.

Homosexual Activity

Usually the pair of children engaging in such sexual activity and very discreet and not discovered. If you do discover them, consider whether or not one or both were "asking to be discovered." If the activity takes place where the likelihood of being discovered was real, then probably one partner is feeling guilty, or one feels the other is pressuring him or her in some way to be part of the act. In any event, when you discover them, you should indicate your disapproval. "That just doesn't go." Then increase your supervision of them when they are together to reduce the opportunity for them to repeat the act. Rarely should the relationship be disrupted if they are of the same age. However, if there is two or three years' difference in their ages, the relationship could be detrimental and probably should be broken up. Almost invariably the older child is pressuring the younger.

If the peer pair is discovered, the worst thing that can happen is for their parents or other adults to overact, and to "stamp" the child's identity as a homosexual, or to engender a sense of guilt with lasting effect. The adolescent experiments with many personalities—and *needs* to do so. He or she needs the freedom to make his choice and not have his environment stick him with any particular one that he experiments with.

Conditions For Homosexuality

Parents who consider it important to be aware of which conditions are known to correlate with homosexuality that persists into adulthood should pay attention to these three that are found in the relationships between a child and his or her parents. One of the relationship patterns is the systematic treatment of a child as though he or she were of the opposite sex, i.e., cross-dressing or being given toys or engaging in activities more appropriate to the opposite sex. He or she concludes from observation that siblings of the opposite sex are favored. In short, if he or she perceives parents rejecting the sex role, the child may reject it, too.

Another pattern is a child who is unable to identify with the parent of the same sex. If the parent is too punitive, the child will come to fear the sex role of the parent as much as the parent. If the parent is psychologically ignoring, unloving, and cold, the child can never want to be like him or her. If the parent is too weak and ineffectual in dealing with others, the child can never want to be like him or her.

A third pattern is a child unable to trust the parent of the opposite sex. If the parent is so emotionally erratic that the child cannot predict his or her emotional response, then the parent cannot be trusted; or similarly if the parent is too seductive.

Seductive Behavior with a Child

A parent is seductive with a child via the emotional tone that typically accompanies such actions as chronic, frequent tickling, riding "horsey," bathing, etc. Bed-sharing and the deliberate immodesty of the parent while dressing or with bathroom functions are other ways. A secretive, confidential relationship implying that the other parent does not care or is just not "in the know" is very seductive.

Seductiveness also usually tends to disrupt the child's peer relationships because it is engulfing and intrusive. The child is not free to develop on his own; everything is tinged with how this potential act would affect the special seductive relationship with the parent. The child also has the definite feeling that something else, a vague something else, is expected of him; something is missing in the relationship to make it complete, to fulfill the parent's need. Analysis of adults shows the vague something to be the sex act itself. The child, however, is aware that that something is something he could not provide. The parent is expecting too much. The detrimental effects in adult life might include impotence (frigidity), inferiority, inability to trust the opposite sex, and fear of competition. It also predisposes the individual to need a triangular situation, at least psychologically, in most all relationships.

Children, even very young children, understand the concept of love; it is an emotion they experience. Sexual feelings should be linked to love feelings for the child. Later, the sexual feelings have to be limited only to certain love objects, and this limiting is part of the struggle of the three- to six-year-old. Unless the sexual feelings are linked primarily with love, the child may link them with aggression or manliness or womanliness, and thus the frequency of intercourse and the number of different partners "conquered" will be more important than the felt relationship to the partner.

Children should see acts of affection between their parents, such as an embrace, hug, or kiss. But they should not be exposed to parental emotions of deep passion and hence certainly not intercourse itself. Thus, precautions should be taken to prevent accidental exposure. They should also, at times, hear disagreements between their parents. It is permissible to be angry and to express it in the love relationship, but children should never overhear violent arguments. Neither should they ever experience fear for their security from a parental argument, nor should they ever hear threats of leaving or divorce. As the child matures physically, so should his or her capacity to experience an ever-widening range of feelings and the capacity to control the expression of those feelings.

Influences

The wide range of influences on children are seldom as unilateral as we have indicated. Our discussion has largely described the influence of one parent modified by the influences of the other parent, grandparents, aunts, uncles, and even adult neighbors who have taken special interest in the child. Although peers will likely be the greatest source of information and misinformation for a curious child, the adults are more likely to be trusted as accurate sources, and to be studied for cues as to how to feel about growing into adult sexual roles. Thus, all of these people play important parts in influencing the child.

Generally speaking, the amount of influence each adult wields is proportional to the closeness the child feels to that person, the love and admiration the child holds for him or her, the strength of that person's personality, and the amount of quality time that person spends with the child. Any adult may essentially diminish this influence through chronic hostility or indifference. Then the child will not want to be like that person, and will actively try to reduce that person's influence, even discouraging that adult's influence in other aspects of the child's life space.

Modulating influences include boys' and girls' exposure to others in positions of respect and guidance. Participating in groups such as scouts, church camps, sports teams, music programs, and tutoring are but a few examples. Exposure to others outside the immediate family provides more opportunities for the child to observe, evaluate, and possibly choose to emulate the qualities he or she admires—even to seek out discussions for expressing concerns and curiosities.

Influences are reinforced and augmented by others if there is congruence—consistency, predictability, and lack of hypocrisy. In general, every influence will tend to move the child toward the center of the dominant cultural mores. Parents can and should be quite important in a child's development of sexual attitudes, but the community will inevitably play a critical role.

It takes a village to raise a (normal) *child.*

And as a normal child gradually takes charge of shepherding himself or herself toward adulthood, you as a parent or other loving adult must remember to be available and accessible, to encourage and recognize those moments when you can make a difference. Remember, whether you are the one who spots the right opportunity, or the child comes to you ready to talk, there is always but one best way to discuss sex:

Frankly.

About the Authors:
Highlights

- From 1964 through 1968, Drs. Marshall L. and Marguerite R. Shearer gave sex lectures, on invitation, to sororities and fraternities and other housing units on the campus of the University of Michigan. During that period they were booked once a week for entire academic years. These talks continued during 1969-70 as well, but to larger audiences. During that time Marshall was on the faculty in the Department of Psychiatry at the University of Michigan School of Medicine, and Marguerite was a physician at the University Health Service.

- In 1970, they were recruited by Dr. Masters and Mrs. Johnson as clinical and research associates. They saw a third of their patients with sexual inadequacies as a therapy team, and were paired with Dr. Masters, Mrs. Johnson, and other staff members for their other patients. In addition, Marshall was responsible for developing the curriculum and doing the initial training for professionals in regard to the foundation's newly described treatment for sexual inadequacies. Marguerite was in charge of the infertility clinic.

- In 1972 they returned to Michigan and continued doing sex therapy, jointly for a while, then Marshall on his own. Marguerite used many of the same principles in her day-to-day family medical practice, including obstetrics and gynecology.

- From 1973 to 1996, the Shearers wrote a sex-help column, answering readers' questions for the *Detroit Free Press,* which was also distributed over the Knight-Ridder wire.

- Marshall is a Board Diplomat of the American Association of Sex Educators, Counselors, and Therapists (AASECT). He is also Board certified in both Psychiatry and Child Psychiatry. Marguerite is Board certified in Family Medicine and also in Medical Management.

- Marshall and Marguerite have been married since 1961, the only marriage for each of them. They have three adult children.

www.DocShearer.com

www.FreshInkGroup.com

About the Authors:
Expanded Narrative

Marshall L. Shearer earned his medical doctor's degree from the Medical College of South Carolina in 1958. After a general rotating internship, he came to the University of Michigan for psychiatric training. He met Marguerite Raft when she was a senior medical student at the University of Michigan. They married in June, 1961, after Marguerite had completed her general rotating internship at Washington DC General Hospital.

Marguerite took a year of advanced training in internal medicine at Wayne County General Hospital in Eloise, Michigan, then a year divided between obstetrics gynecology and surgery at Women's Hospital of Detroit.

Marshall continued his psychiatric residency, which included a year in research and certification in child psychiatry. For about 18 months in 1962-63, he consulted one day a week with the Michigan Department of Corrections. Part of his responsibility was to do psychiatric evaluations on men who had recently arrived in prison to serve life sentences.

After their marriage, they joined the Bushnell Congregational Church on Southfield Road in Detroit. Marshall taught Sunday school there for one year. Marguerite and Marshall were recruited by the Minister to Youth, William Straight, to be resource physicians for a sex education program sponsored by the church and put on by Mrs. and Mr. Ventor. The program was divided between the junior-high and high-school students; the pupils in each group were both male and female.

The following year, the Shearers moved to Dexter, Michigan. Marshall completed his psychiatric training and joined the University of Michigan School of Medicine faculty full time, first as an Instructor, then later as an Assistant Professor.

Marguerite took a position as a physician at the University of Michigan Student Health Service, where she saw many coeds as patients. She soon became aware of the problems that many college students were facing in regard to sexual issues, particularly after the university eliminated housemothers and made dormitories coed. She was the first physician at the Student Health Service to prescribe contraceptives to students.

Marguerite saw a number of female students who had engaged in intercourse without being fully cognizant of what was happening, sometimes resulting in unwanted pregnancies. She was alarmed by some of the stories related by women who had elected to have abortions, which was illegal in those years. They included being separated from the psychological support of people they trusted, sometimes even being blindfolded and led down an alley where the procedure was to be done by a complete stranger. Some women reported hearing rodents scurrying around. Marguerite was further alarmed by the potential for injury to the women's reproductive systems and for life-threatening infections.

This led Marguerite and Marshall to volunteer to give sex education lectures, on request, to students living in housing units at the University of Michigan.

Marshall became a diplomat of the American Board of Neurology and Psychiatry in Psychiatry, and later of the same Board in Child Psychiatry. Marguerite became a Diplomat of the American Board of Family Medicine and, later, Medical Management.

At Children's Psychiatric Hospital at the University of Michigan as Assistant In-Patient Director, Marshall began working with couples in regard to their hospitalized children. He also consulted for Dr. Hazel Turner of the Ann Arbor Public Schools for one-half day each week from 1965–69.

Marshall conceived the idea of bringing a dog into the hospital, believing that it would have a therapeutic effect on patients ages 5 or 6, up to 12. They could relate to the dog with a "fresh slate," presumably with little or no emotional hold-over from their pasts.

The dog would respond to the children's affection, and would give the kids something to love without making demands on them. The affection returned by the dog would be directly proportional to the affection it received. This experiment was supported by Marshall's section chief, Dr. Stuart Finch, and the Department of Psychiatry chair, Dr. Raymond Waggoner. With the assistance of Mr. Cleveland, of Hospital Administration, the request was approved.

Some time later, the dog got loose while being exercised on the hospital grounds, and subsequently had puppies. This created some stir— not so much with the children or the child-care workers, but somewhat with the nurses and quite a bit with some of the psychiatric residents who struggled with how to deal with the issue and how to give sex education to their young patients and support staff. The experience with the dog in the hospital was published by Elizabeth Yates, one of the child-care staff.[1]

Dr. Raymond Waggoner was also a member of the Board of Directors of Masters and Johnson Institute. At that time the organization was known as the Reproductive Biological Research Foundation. The RBRF had just completed its study of the treatment of sexual dysfunction and was interested in hiring a medical couple who were comfortable talking about sex. They also wanted a psychiatrist and someone from academia who had experience in teaching. Dr. Waggoner recruited Marshall and Marguerite.

While with Masters and Johnson, Marguerite and Marshall each carried a load of three new patients every two weeks. One-third of Marguerite's cases were with Dr. Masters, one-third with Dr. Spitz, and one-third with Marshall. Marguerite also was responsible for the RBRF Foundation's infertility clinic. Marshall's caseload was similarly divided. In addition to treating patients, he

---

[1] Elizabeth Yates: *Skeezer, Dog with a Mission*, Harvey House, Inc., Irvington-on-Hudson, New York, 1973

was responsible for developing a curriculum with Mrs. Johnson, and for teaching the first group of professionals.

Upon their return to Michigan, Marguerite and Marshall opened a joint sexual counseling practice. Marshall continued with his general psychiatric practice and had a clinical assignment at the University of Michigan as Associate Professor of Psychiatry. Marguerite practiced Family Medicine.

Marguerite was elected president of the Washtenaw County Medical Society in 1980. In 1983, she was the first woman elected to the Board of Directors of the Michigan State Medical Society. She was on the Michigan Delegation to the American Medical Association from 1990 until 2002.

Together, the Shearers have 57 years working extensively with heterosexual and gay couples and individuals in relationships. They have taken thousands of detailed sexual histories on both men and women.

Marguerite R. Shearer is now an active member of the First Unitarian Universalist Church of Ann Arbor, Michigan. Marshall L. Shearer passed away in 2015 at the age of 82. He left his last project, a manuscript titled *Toward Interfaith Harmony*, to be published posthumously. □

www.DocShearer.com

www.FreshInkGroup.com

Also by The Doctors Shearer!

MAXIMIZING HAPPINESS THROUGH INTIMATE COMMUNICATION

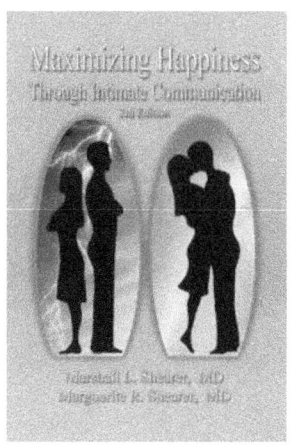

Self-Help Relationship Advice, Marriage Solutions, Couples Therapy, Great Sex, & More!

True love is nurtured in the conviction that you both value your partner's happiness as much as your own, but achieving such confidence in any relationship is a challenge, even for the most committed. No matter what lifestyle you pursue together, it's through honest communication that you will learn to protect yourselves and each other, to shed the encumbrances of clutter and noise as you propel your own unique Spiral of Love to exhilarating new heights.

From finding your soulmate through growing old together, *Maximizing Happiness Through Intimate Communication* lays out a complete system with everyday examples, simply explaining relationship dynamics like persistent problems, the transformation of hurts, concepts of time, components of anger, addictions, turning work into play, protecting vulnerability, reinforcing trust, sexual communication, and the neverending stages of love's spiral.

Don't be discouraged by media-packaged gimmicks and the one-size-fits-all advice from self-help gurus. Become the experts of your own relationship, and discover the best of growing yourselves that ultimate, most meaningful love.

www.FreshInkGroup.com

ISBN: 978-1-936442-01-0

Also by Marshall L. Shearer, MD!

MY LIFE AND SPIRITUAL JOURNEY

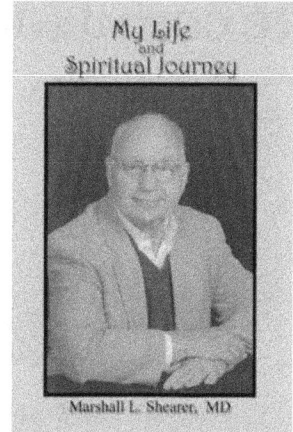

From Tragedy to Acceptance, How One Atheist Looked Beyond Doctrines To Integrate Our World's Religions

The child of a military family, young Marshall Shearer dealt with personal tragedy by formulating poignant questions that led to contradictory and unsatisfactory religion-based explanations. He never stopped seeking answers, even as he has enjoyed a wonderful life: medical school, loving marriage, beautiful family, and a distinguished career dedicated to helping people learn to live happily, to embrace others, and to cherish life. Through it all, he persisted as a student of the world's religions, asking new and ever-more sophisticated questions and finding answers we can all accept, from atheists to the most devout. Having developed his own unique perspective for understanding our place in the world, he continues to share his vision through books ranging from how to grow successful relationships to advocating bold new ways to achieve harmony among all religions. In *My Life and Spiritual Journey*, Dr. Shearer tells us his own story, the intimate perspective of one determined man who refuses to compromise in his quest to discover the acceptance we all seek and deserve.

www.FreshInkGroup.com

ISBN: 978-1-936442-02-7

BEEN THERE, NOTED THAT:

Essays in Celebration of Life

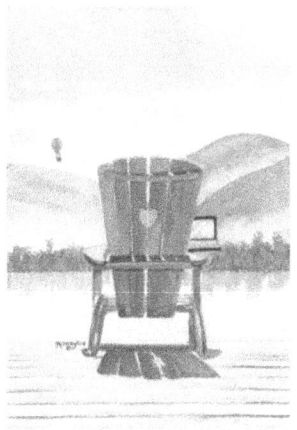

**Observations, Inspiration, Remembrance,
& Noteworthies To Share**

By Stephen Geez

The simple lives of everyday people in a mundane world prove extraordinary in this collection of 54 personal-experience essays by novelist Stephen Geez. The eclectic mix of memoir, commentary, humor, and appreciation covers a wide range of topics, each beautifully illustrated by artists and photographers from the Fresh Ink Group. Geez catches what many of us miss, then considers how we might all share the most poignant of lessons. *Been There, Noted That* aims to reveal who we are, examine where we've been, and discover what we dare strive to become.

www.FreshInkGroup.com

ISBN: 978-978-1-936442-05-8

www.ingramcontent.com/pod-product-compliance
Lightning Source LLC
Chambersburg PA
CBHW020001050426
42450CB00005B/274